THE WHOLE FOOD PREGNANCY PLAN

EAT CLEAN & FEEL GOOD WITH
COMPLETE NUTRITION

AIMEE ARISTOTELOUS
foreword by DR. KENNETH AKEY

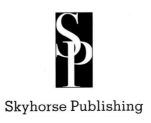

Skyhorse Publishing

Skyhorse Publishing books may be purchased in bulk at special discounts for sales promotion, corporate gifts, fund-raising, or educational purposes. Special editions can also be created to specifications. For details, contact the Special Sales Department, Skyhorse Publishing, 307 West 36th Street, 11th Floor, New York, NY 10018 or info@skyhorsepublishing.com.

Skyhorse® and Skyhorse Publishing® are registered trademarks of Skyhorse Publishing, Inc.®, a Delaware corporation.

Visit our website at www.skyhorsepublishing.com.

10 9 8 7 6 5 4 3 2 1

Library of Congress Cataloging-in-Publication Data available on file.

Cover design by David Ter-Avanesyan
Cover photo from Shutterstock

Print ISBN: 978-1-5107-6867-3
Ebook ISBN: 978-1-5107-7055-3

Printed in China

*For the two in my life who made me a mom, Richard and Alex,
and for my own mom and dad, Norma and Steve.*

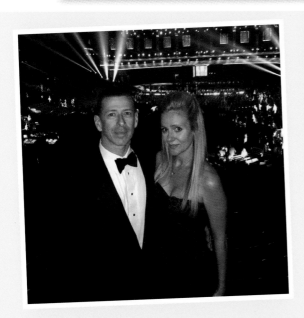

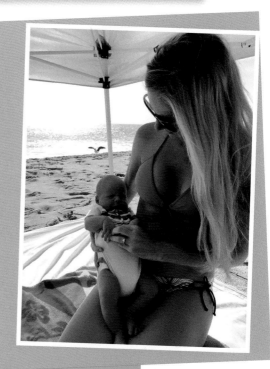

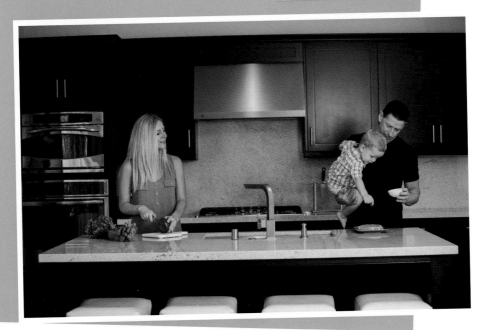

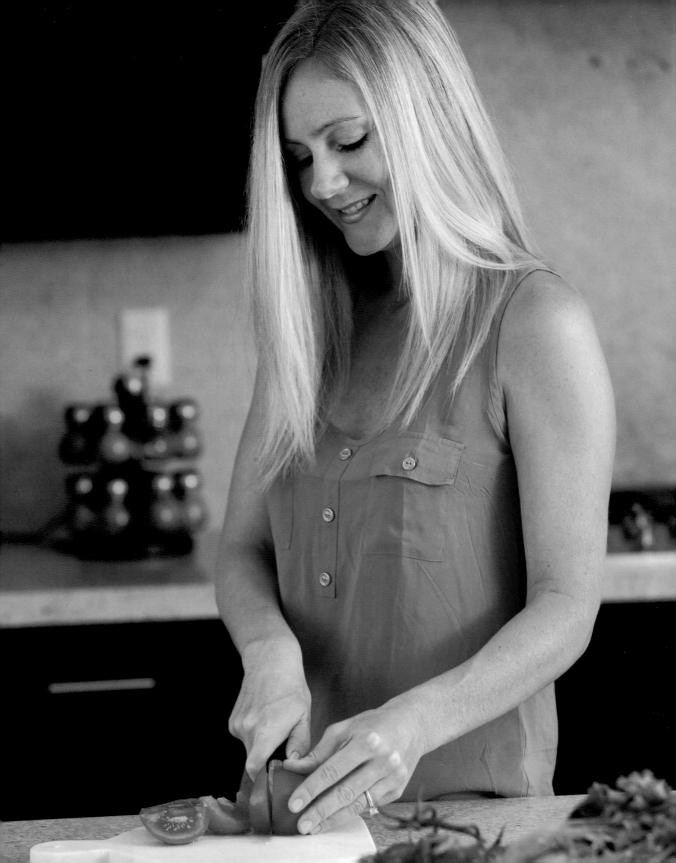

Table of Contents

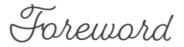

Foreword

By Dr. Kenneth Akey, MD

Who will sound the alarm? Who will stand up and unabashedly speak the truth regarding our children's and family's health? It is an obvious fact that our opulent, overindulgent society is sadly unhealthy. Why? Many very bright minds with vast resources are supposedly working together for the good of our precious children. And there is so much interest and passion to help.

Fortunately, there are voices—authors and researchers today actively looking for answers. There are many books on the shelves about nutrition and health. Thank God for these people. *Un*fortunately, many of these books are mainly interested in weight loss, not true good health.

Aimee Aristotelous is authentically passionate about the health of the pregnant mother and pre- and post-delivery infant. She is a certified nutritionist and the amazing mom of little Alexander, both of whom I have the privilege of knowing as their pediatrician. I love spending time

with Aimee, her hubby Richard, and little Alex during their well checkups. At two years old, Alex has not had one sick visit—strangest thing!?

Aimee is a committed advocate of healthy families. She has written and presented on numerous nutrition topics via social media, television, and live presentations. It is a pleasure and an honor to be a part of her book. I speak about nutrition with every patient I see, just as Aimee does with her clients and contacts. Not to be too simplistic, but nutrition is what health is all about.

Almost every book I have ever read about health, nutrition, or preventive medicine has included a long list of chronic, extremely common medical conditions. I'll only list the several that I see every day: toxic substances in our environment, food additives, sweeteners, fast food, junk food, and over-medication all have been associated with the emergence of new dangers and tragic illnesses, including speech delays, attention deficit hyperactivity disorder (ADHD), allergies, asthma, irritable bowel syndrome (IBS), celiac disease, gluten sensitivity, type 2 diabetes, and obesity. These are horrible conditions and diseases that become more prevalent every day.

What can you, an expectant mother or new parent, do? You can read about nutrition in books and on the internet, buy food from reputable sources, or even grow some of your own vegetables and fruits. You can follow people like Aimee and her contributors on Facebook and other social media. You can always be learning and looking for new information. My point, and the point of *The Whole Food Pregnancy Plan*, is to be curious, investigate, read ingredient labels, be wary and distrustful of processed foods, be proactive, and search out a healthy lifestyle. Speak louder than the processed food industry and fast food companies and don't compromise your family's health.

Thanks to Aimee and her contributors for providing the truth about how to have a healthy pregnancy and baby through pure and natural nutrition. I encourage you to take heart and dive into the following pages with excitement, and also with a deep sense of urgency. Good reading, good health, and God bless!

Introduction

Yes, you can have a healthy, gluten-free pregnancy! Whether you have celiac disease, Non-Celiac Gluten Sensitivity (NCGS) or you just feel better when avoiding gluten, *The Whole Food Pregnancy Plan* is a safe and nutritionally superior gluten-free guide that helps expecting and postpartum women achieve ideal health and weight during pregnancy and beyond. Implementing philosophies of current, highly-effective gluten-free nutrition trends that, until now, have not been fully introduced to the prenatal and postpartum populations, *The Whole Food Pregnancy Plan* offers a detailed dietary regimen that is based on whole and unprocessed foods, low-glycemic carbohydrates, quality proteins, and essential fats.

This book is a nutrition education guide, recipe book, and meal planner all in one! Whether you are non-vegan or vegan, this book is for you as it caters to both nutrition lifestyles, containing information and recipes which include both animal- and plant-based proteins. It also provides special instruction for each stage of pregnancy, including the first, second, and third trimesters, as well as the "fourth trimester" of postpartum weight loss and nursing. Furthermore, it will inform you about deceptive marketing strategies and harmful ingredients used by commercial baby food manufacturers, and advise how to provide the most beneficial nutrition for your infant.

The recipes and meal plans found throughout *The Whole Food Pregnancy Plan* vary with regard to dietary lifestyles, stages of pregnancy, trimester-specific dietary needs, pregnancy-related conditions, and lengths of preparation/cooking time. Since not everyone enjoys cooking or has the time to spend in the kitchen, the meal plans and recipes fluctuate in terms of simplicity and time. You will find that many of the meal plans contain basic instructions as opposed to detailed recipes for the sake of ease and time constraints. If you are someone who wants to get a bit more adventurous in the kitchen, I have more than 100 detailed recipes for you!

In addition to being a recipe book and meal planner, *The Whole Food Pregnancy Plan* provides a broad spectrum of nutrition information regarding required vitamins and minerals, as well as superior forms of fats, proteins, and carbohydrates. You will learn about the superstar nutrients needed during preconception and each trimester of pregnancy, as well as how to obtain them. If you're wondering how you will meet your fiber and folic acid requirements while avoiding gluten, I'll show you a variety of exceptional, nutrient-dense options which boast naturally occurring nutrients as opposed to fortified versions that are found in most commercially-made gluten-containing foods.

I wrote this book to show you how to have an amazingly healthy, enjoyable, and active gluten-free pregnancy, the same way I did! Eliminating gluten from your diet doesn't have to mean eliminating vital nutrients needed for your pregnancy. In fact, refraining from eating gluten-foods will dramatically lessen the amount of processed, high-glycemic carbohydrates you consume, which will have beneficial effects on you and your baby. Congratulations and welcome to your whole pregnancy journey!

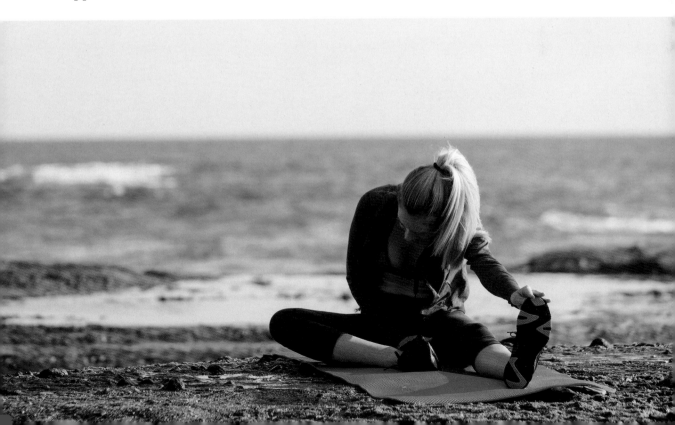

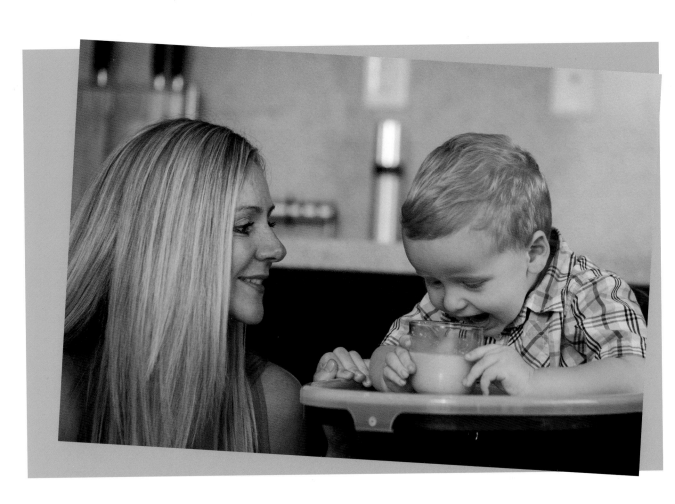

Chapter 1
Pregnancy Nutrition Recommendations Today

On December 11, 2014, I got the big news at my doctor's office—I was expecting! I was given a large goody bag filled with everything from prenatal vitamin samples to umbilical cord blood banking service pamphlets. As a certified nutritionist, I naturally gravitated toward the packet of nutrition information, which covered topics such as proper weight gain during pregnancy, how to avoid gestational diabetes, and foods one should eat to benefit mother and baby. The pamphlet, a generic one which most likely circulates through thousands of doctors' offices, listed the following as a daily guide for "good nutrition during pregnancy."

One may look at these recommendations and nod at the fact that they seem "normal" for today's standards and yes, they are normal; however, they are extremely faulty and actually contribute to serious medical conditions that run rampant in today's population of pregnant women, such as gestational diabetes and excessive weight gain. Let's take this recommended daily intake of food and break it down into macro-nutrients (carbohydrates, protein, fat) as well as sugar so we can get a better understanding of the implications of these suggested foods.

As you can see, this suggested example of one day of "healthy food" results in 100 grams of sugar, as well as an abundance of carbohydrates from processed gluten-foods. To put it into perspective, this is

Daily Recommended Foods and Servings
2 slices of bread
1 cup of cereal
1½ cups of pasta
2½ cups of vegetables
2 cups of fruit or fruit juice
5 ounces of meat, poultry, fish, beans, eggs, or nuts
3 cups of milk

FOOD	CARBOHYDRATES	PROTEIN	FAT	SUGAR
Whole Wheat Bread (2 Slices)	24g	8g	2g	4g
Whole Grain Cereal (1 Cup)	29g	3g	2g	7g
Whole Wheat Pasta (1½ Cups)	54g	11g	2g	2g
Broccoli (1 Cup)	9g	3g	0g	2g
Carrots (1½ Cups)	12g	2g	0g	9g
Sliced Banana (1 Cup)	34g	2g	0g	18g
Orange Juice (1 Cup)	26g	2g	0g	22g
Chicken (5 Ounces)	0g	30g	2g	0g
2% Milk (3 Cups)	36g	24g	15g	36g
TOTALS	224g	85g	23g	**100 g**

equivalent to eating ten glazed donuts in one day! One may say that sugars from the above listed foods are different than refined sugar—unfortunately, your body is negatively affected by too much sugar, whether it comes from a refined or natural source. Another possible argument is that these foods do offer a variety of nutritional benefits (unlike ten glazed donuts), thus justifying the sugar and carbohydrate intake. I will explain in later chapters how to get twice the nutrients that this typical plan offers, while consuming less than half the sugar, and no high-glycemic, gluten-containing carbohydrates (your carbs will come from different sources)!

Why is it so important that we reduce sugar and high-glycemic carbohydrate intake? According to the Center for Disease Control, gestational diabetes affects up to ten percent of all pregnant women. Gestational diabetes occurs around the twenty-fourth week of pregnancy and is a result of the placenta releasing hormones that make it difficult for the mother's body to create and use insulin. Insulin is needed to balance blood sugar levels; if you don't make and use enough insulin, then sugar or glucose builds up in your blood. Not only is this dangerous to the mother, it can also negatively affect the baby as the excess glucose crosses the placenta, resulting in high sugar levels for the baby. The baby's pancreas will work overtime to combat the extra glucose which crosses the placenta by releasing insulin. Babies born to mothers with gestational diabetes are at higher risk of growing into children and adults who develop type II diabetes and obesity.[1]

Conditions such as gestational diabetes put the mother at risk as well. According to the World Health Organization, around twenty-eight women die in the United States for every 100,000 births. This number has more than doubled since 1990, resulting in the United States being the only developed country that has a maternal mortality rate that is on the rise.[2] This is due to a plethora of issues that face pregnant women, including increased rates of obesity, cardiovascular disease, and diabetes. What do all of these conditions have in common? It is possible to combat and regulate them through diet alone. Unfortunately, the outdated nutrition recommendations made by the literature provided in the offices of many OB-GYNs may actually cause these conditions—not prevent them!

In addition to nutrition recommendations given in pamphlets that I received from my doctor, I began to explore the information in popular pregnancy nutrition books as well. I came across a best-selling pregnancy nutrition book that boasts examples of daily menus including the sample shown on the next page. Once again, I'll break this sample menu down so we can understand how many grams of sugar one will consume when following this advice.

Going back to the comparison of sugar in glazed donuts, this day of "healthy food" equates to thirteen donuts! After realizing that these types of recommendations are the primary sources of information for pregnant women, I decided to research titles written by widely popular medical organizations to see if their advice aligned with these faulty guidelines. To no surprise, they, too recommend high-sugar, high-carbohydrate, gluten-filled diets which are disguised as "healthy foods."

1   Sharon Herring and Emily Oken, "Obesity and Diabetes in Mothers and Their Children: Can We Stop the Intergenerational Cycle?" NCBI, February 01, 2011, accessed September 04, 2017, https://www.ncbi.nlm.nih.gov/pmc/articles/PMC3191112/pdf/nihms327612.pdf.

2   "Global, regional, and national levels of maternal mortality, 1990–2015: a systematic analysis for the Global Burden of Disease Study 2015," NCBI, October 08, 2016, accessed September 04, 2017, https://www.ncbi.nlm.nih.gov/pubmed/?term=GBD%202015%20Maternal%20Mortality%20Collaborators%5BCorporate%20Author%5D

Breakfast

1 cup fortified whole grain breakfast cereal
1 cup reduced-fat (2%) milk
1 slice whole wheat bread, toasted
1 tablespoon peanut butter
½ cup calcium-fortified orange juice

Lunch

1 whole wheat pita
½ cup hummus
5 cherry tomatoes, 4 cucumber slices, and 1 cup mixed greens with 1 tablespoon light salad dressing
1 peach

Snack

1 granola bar
1 cup low-fat blueberry yogurt

Dinner

4 ounces store-bought roasted chicken breast
1 medium size baked potato
2 tablespoons reduced-fat sour cream
½ cup broccoli florets
¾ cup coleslaw
1 cup reduced-fat 2% milk
½ cup frozen low-fat vanilla yogurt

FOOD	SUGAR
Whole Grain Cereal (1 Cup)	7 grams
2% Milk (1 Cup)	12 grams
Whole Wheat Bread (1 Slice)	2 grams
Peanut Butter (1 Tablespoon)	1 gram
Orange Juice (½ Cup)	12 grams
Whole Wheat Pita (1 Piece)	1 gram
Hummus (½ Cup)	0 grams
Cherry Tomatoes (5)	3 grams
Cucumber Slices (4)	0 grams
Mixed Greens (1 Cup)	0 grams
Light Salad Dressing (1 Teaspoon)	1 gram
Peach (1)	13 grams

Granola Bar (1)	10 grams
Low-fat Blueberry Yogurt (1 Cup)	26 grams
Chicken Breast (4 Ounces)	0 grams
Baked Potato (1 Medium)	2 grams
Reduced Fat Sour Cream (2 Tablespoons)	0 grams
Broccoli Florets (½ Cup)	1 gram
Coleslaw (¾ Cup)	10 grams
2% Milk (1 Cup)	12 grams
Frozen Low-fat Vanilla Yogurt (1/2 Cup)	17 grams
TOTAL	130 grams

One widely relied-upon organization in particular even stated that pregnant women should "stay away from fat such as avocado," despite the fact that avocado is a pregnancy super-food as the growing fetus thrives on healthy fats for brain development (I'll get into that in later chapters)!

I decided to write *The Whole Food Pregnancy Plan* because the current nutrition recommendations for pregnant women are still based on old frameworks such as the food pyramid from the 1970s. After seeing the advice that is offered in several literary sources and in doctors' offices, it's no wonder that millions of pregnant women are suffering from diet-related conditions despite the fact that they are, most likely, following the advice given to them by their doctors and nutritionists. I applied my own research to create my own case study during my pregnancy and I will share in the following chapters the gluten-free nutrition regimen that resulted in a twenty-five-pound weight gain and nine-pound, twelve-ounce healthy baby boy. Despite the fact that I was a woman of "advanced maternal age" which implies that I would be more susceptible to conditions like gestational diabetes, hypertension, and preeclampsia, my blood sugar levels and blood pressure remained in perfect ranges. I had a completely natural, drug-free child birth and returned to my pre-pregnancy weight before my six-week postpartum check-up—and you can do the same!

Chapter 2
The Whole Food Pregnancy Principles

Today's food supply is quite different than the one our ancestors knew. The primary philosophy of *The Whole Food Pregnancy Plan* is to get back to the basics and eat real food. Eating whole foods that are nutrient dense, unprocessed, and organic (when available) is ideal for the expectant mother and growing baby. Whether you are vegan, vegetarian, or a meat eater, *The Whole Food Pregnancy Plan* will help you have your healthiest pregnancy possible—if followed properly, you'll gain an appropriate amount of weight, have amazing energy, and possibly combat that pesky morning sickness. The most important benefit is you will obtain ideal nutrition for yourself and your baby. Below are the principles you will be following throughout your whole pregnancy:

Principle ① Focus on nutrient-dense foods as opposed to synthetic vitamins.

You will learn how to eat a balanced diet of whole foods, providing the most substantial nutrient intake without the need to supplement with synthetic, hard-to-absorb commercial vitamins. Synthetic vitamins provide a false security for many women when they are expecting which can lead to consuming foods that are void of nutrition while relying on obtaining adequate nutrients from a supplement alone. In coming chapters, I will reference a variety of nutrient-dense foods that are catered to different nutrition lifestyles.

Principle ② Be mindful of your calorie intake.

Due to increased hormones, our senses increase during pregnancy and this can make the taste and smell of some foods absolutely euphoric which may lead some to eat out of pure pleasure. Pregnant women actually do not need as many calories as the old saying "eating for two" implies. In fact, you will not need any additional calories at all in your first trimester and only a few hundred extra in subsequent trimesters if carrying a singleton. Being mindful of your calorie intake means to eat when you are

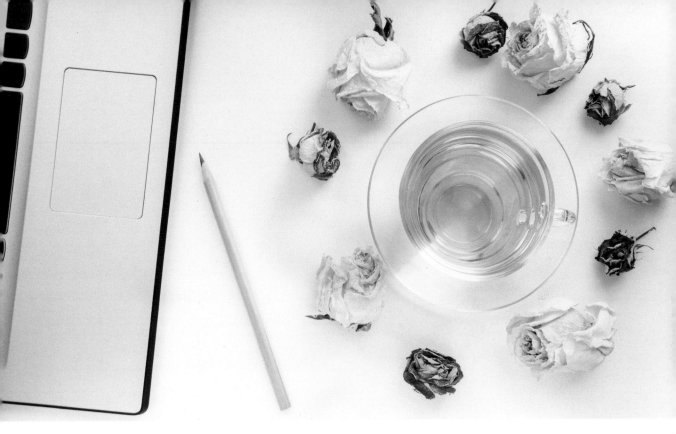

hungry and stop when you are content but not overly full.

Principle ③ Eat an abundance of healthy fats.

Past research has demonized the consumption of fats and the popular misconception that all fat is bad still remains in many prenatal nutrition sources despite the fact that recent studies have shown a correlation between healthy fat consumption during pregnancy with proper fetal brain and eye development.[3]

These healthy, omega-3 fatty acids can be consumed from foods such as low-mercury fish (or even from fish oil supplements), walnuts, egg yolks, and seaweed. You will learn the difference between a variety of fats in coming chapters, as well as the many sources you can find them in.

Principle ④ Consume more quality proteins.

Several nutrition books and resources still recommend as little as forty-five grams of protein per day for the pregnant woman

---

3   J. Coletta, S. Bell, and A. Roman, "Omega-3 Fatty Acids and Pregnancy," NCBI, October 2010, accessed September 10, 2017, https://www.ncbi.nlm.nih.gov/pmc/articles/PMC3046737/#__ffn_sect.

despite the fact that the amino acids found in protein are the building blocks of your baby's cells and tissues. According to the Institute of Medicine, expectant mothers should eat at least seventy-one grams of protein per day. Furthermore, the American Pregnancy Association recommends consuming as much as 100 grams of protein per day. The faulty yet popular recommendation of forty-five grams of protein per day results in a diet that consists of only nine percent protein based on a 2,000-calorie diet. *The Whole Food Pregnancy Plan* will provide the proper types and amounts of protein to be consumed for a healthy pregnancy.

Principle ⑤ Limit or eliminate cow's milk.

Yes, your doctor has probably recommended 2–3 servings of cow's milk per day due to the fact that it has calcium. Unfortunately, commercial cow's milk can contain large amounts of estrogens and progesterone which may not be ideal for human consumption.[4] Some studies are suggesting that intake

of commercial cow's milk may be cause for concern to the general public and more research may be needed.[5] Now, if you like a little bit of creamer in your tea or a serving of Greek yogurt or kefir (great sources of probiotics), that's one thing, but consistently high intake of dairy may be best to be avoided. You will consume a variety of calcium sources (provided in later chapters) that are most beneficial to mother and growing baby as they boast a multitude of other nutrients in addition to bioavailable calcium.

Principle ⑥ Restrict processed foods.

Yes, it may happen (and it may happen more than once)—you could have a craving for something out of a box! You don't have to eat perfectly 100 percent of the time to have a healthy pregnancy (I will explain the "90/10 rule" later in this chapter), but processed foods cannot be relied upon as a normal staple in your food regimen. Most processed foods are high in sugar, carbohydrates, additives, and preservatives, and they do not offer naturally occurring

---

4   K. Mayurama, T. Oshima, and K. Ohyama, "Exposure to exogenous estrogen through intake of commercial milk produced from pregnant cows," NCBI, February 2010, accessed September 10, 2017, https://www.ncbi.nlm.nih.gov/pubmed/19496976.

5   H. Malekinejad and A. Rezabakhsh, "Hormones in Dairy Foods and Their Impact on Public Health—A Narrative Review Article," Hormones in Dairy Foods and Their Impact on Public Health—A Narrative Review Article, June 2015, accessed September 10, 2017, https://www.ncbi.nlm.nih.gov/pmc/articles/PMC4524299/.

nutrients that are imperative to your growing baby.

Principle ⑦ Choose gluten-free, low-glycemic foods as a primary carbohydrate source.

The Glycemic Index is a measurement tool used to gauge how carbohydrate-containing foods affect blood sugar levels. Coincidentally, gluten selections such as bread, crackers, pasta, and cereals, are high-glycemic, causing dramatic rises and dips in blood sugar levels which can lead to cravings, fatigue, and gestational diabetes. Low-glycemic carbohydrate choices such as green vegetables, berries, beans, and quinoa help to maintain even blood sugar levels and satiety by breaking down into glucose at a much slower rate. In addition, the low-glycemic carbohydrates mentioned above are minimally processed and contain a variety of naturally occurring, bioavailable vitamins and minerals as opposed to the fortified, synthetic nutrients found in their high-glycemic counterparts.

You may be wondering what gluten is and why it may be beneficial to avoid gluten-containing foods. Gluten is a substance present in grains, including wheat, barley, and rye, that is responsible for the elastic texture of dough; it causes

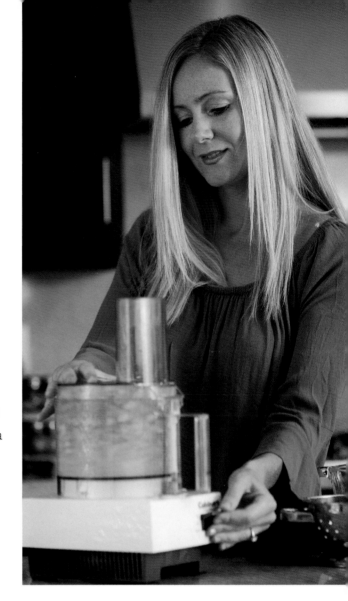

illness in people with celiac disease. Celiac disease is a severe autoimmune condition that results in an immune response that attacks the small intestine after ingestion of gluten-containing foods. This phenomenon can lead to impaired function of the small intestine, resulting in the inability to absorb nutrients from foods.

This is for every man and woman that is at all considering starting a family at any time in their life. My initial advice to you is this: get tested for celiac disease as soon as possible. Ideally, every woman, child, and man in the world would be tested as soon as possible to identify which 30–50 percent of the population carries the main genes for celiac, HLA-DQ2 and/or HLA-DQ8. If you or your partner are gene carriers for these genes then the first plan of action would be to get properly tested for celiac disease. That can include an antibody test such as a serum celiac panel, a stool test from Enterolab, an Array 3 test from CyrexLabs, and/or an intestinal biopsy. Any antibody test absolutely needs to include a Total IgA and IgG due to the fact that many of the people with celiac disease are IgA deficient which means antibody testing is not useful or accurate because the person is not producing enough IgA necessary to mount an effective immune response due to damage in the intestines. Please keep in mind, one test does not rule celiac disease out; you can have symptoms or not and everyone, world-wide, is at risk of developing celiac disease or NCGS at any age (if you are a gene carrier). Celiac disease, by way of an innate and adaptive immune response to wheat, barley, rye, and contaminated oats, causes damage to the intestines of people that are gene carriers of HLA-DQ2 and/or HLA-DQ8. Carrying these genes predisposes people to having celiac disease if they are exposed to even minute or trace amounts of these grains. The beauty of this information is that if you are a gene carrier and you are never exposed to these grains, then you will never develop celiac disease. If, however, you are a gene carrier, then you can develop celiac disease at any point during your life, provided you are exposed to these grains. If you and your partner are both gene carriers then the chance of your child(ren) carrying these gene increases and the potential to be homozygous, getting genes from each parent or having two copies of the genes associated with celiac disease, thereby increases the risk of developing celiac disease exponentially. Unfortunately, most people are unaware of their genetic status for HLA-DQ2 and/or DQ8, despite the fact that these genes for celiac disease are extremely common worldwide, in every ethnic group, without exception.

—Nadine Grzeskowiak, RN, BSN, CEN

You may be thinking, "I don't have celiac disease so why should I go gluten-free during my pregnancy?" During my own pregnancy, I severely limited gluten, not because I have been diagnosed with celiac disease but because in the past I did show symptoms of Non-Celiac Gluten Sensitivity (migraines, stomach pains, and weight gain, to name a few) leading me to give up regular consumption of gluten-foods back in 2011. If you are someone who suffers from celiac disease or Non-Celiac Gluten Sensitivity (NCGS), or maybe you are wondering if you are at risk, it is critical to take the proper precautions to keep yourself and your family healthy. Even if you have never experienced gluten sensitivity, maybe you just feel better when limiting or eliminating gluten as there are an assortment of implications that come with gluten-containing foods.

As I mentioned in Chapter 1, in the United States, up to ten percent of all pregnant women suffer from gestational diabetes which means that hundreds of thousands of pregnant women will suffer from gestational diabetes this year, in America alone—and this trend is on the rise! Foods (that coincidentally contain gluten) are also high-carbohydrate and high-glycemic which means these foods will raise blood sugar when consumed and the drastic rise in blood sugar resulting from regular consumption of these foods could lead to gestational diabetes, cravings, and excessive weight gain. Pregnant women are especially vulnerable to high-carbohydrate and high-glycemic foods because they produce hormones in the placenta during pregnancy that can result in an excess amount of sugar in the blood to begin with. Enough insulin may be excreted from the pancreas to combat this, but if that fails to happen, blood sugar levels will continue to increase which leads to gestational diabetes. Due to this phenomenon, it is imperative that all pregnant women are mindful of foods that are high in carbohydrates and high on the glycemic index since their insulin resistance may already be elevated through hormonal activity.[6] Coincidentally, these foods also contain gluten, so even if you are not someone who suffers from celiac disease or (NCGS), avoiding gluten will result in avoiding several foods that will raise your blood sugar.

---

6   A. Sonagra, S. Biradar, and J. Murthy, "Normal Pregnancy—A State of Insulin Resistance," Journal of Clinical and Diagnostic Research, November 2014, accessed September 10, 2017, https://www.ncbi.nlm.nih.gov/pmc/articles/PMC4290225/.

Besides gestational diabetes, let's take a look at a few other implications gluten-foods may have on your health while expecting. As many as half of all pregnant women will experience constipation—it's a very common problem! The increase in the hormone progesterone relaxes the muscles in the digestive tract so food ends up moving through the intestines at a slower pace. Gluten (which is Latin for "glue") does not help this situation as its glue-like features may cause the gluten-food to glom onto other foods that are eaten in the same timeframe, hindering suitable digestion which can contribute to constipation.[7] In addition, fighting inflammation in order to support your immune system is imperative while you are expecting and reducing gluten-containing foods may also reduce inflammation.[8]

Another implication of gluten-containing foods is that a considerable amount of non-organic wheat is treated with Monsanto's Roundup which means that many gluten-containing processed

> Even in the absence of celiac disease, glyphosate has been shown to produce intestinal damage or increased permeability of the intestinal wall in humans.
> **—Nadine Grzeskowiak, RN, BSN, CEN**

foods also contain glyphosate, a chemical found in the widely-used weed killer. According to International Agency for Research on Cancer, glyphosate is classified as a "probable carcinogen." Several studies suggest that a "probable carcinogen" is probably not an ideal item to be putting in our bodies when we are growing a baby (or even if we are not growing a baby)! Keep in mind that most non-organic wheat, as well as the multitude of processed foods that contain wheat, have been treated with glyphosate—I'll go more into detail about glyphosate and genetically modified organisms (GMOs) in Chapter 11.

Coincidentally, the majority of foods that contain gluten are also highly processed with detrimental ingredients. They have long shelf lives and contain

---

7   A. Sadeghi, S. Shahrokh, and M. Reza Zali, "An unusual cause of constipation in a patient without any underlying disorders," NCBI, February 19, 2015, accessed September 10, 2017, https://www.ncbi.nlm.nih.gov/pmc/articles/PMC4403030/.

8   K. De Punder and L. Pruimboom, "The Dietary Intake of Wheat and other Cereal Grains and Their Role in Inflammation," NCBI, March 12, 2015, accessed September 10, 2017, https://www.ncbi.nlm.nih.gov/pmc/articles/PMC3705319/#!-po=59.5238.

harmful preservatives as well as other additives that will not contribute to your healthiest pregnancy. Some of these common ingredients that are found in gluten-containing, processed foods include but are not limited to soybean oil, high-fructose corn syrup, and soy lecithin.

The majority of US soybeans are, like non-organic wheat, treated with Monsanto's glyphosate, therefore the widely popular soybean oil that is found in numerous processed foods is also contaminated with the "probable carcinogen." In addition, a high percentage of US corn is also treated with glyphosate so not only does high-fructose corn syrup contain a "probable carcinogen," it is also even sweeter than sugar and we know that excessive sweeteners during pregnancy can be damaging. Soy lecithin is an additive that gives food a smooth texture; the chemical solvent hexane (a neurotoxin) is used to extract oil from the soybeans so traces of hexane will remain in these processed foods. Animal studies have suggested that a relatively small percentage of soy lecithin intake during pregnancy has resulted in unfavorable offspring outcomes such as poor reflexes and behavioral abnormalities.[9] Not only are the above-mentioned unfavorable ingredients found in processed foods for adults, but baby foods contain them as well. I explore these ingredients and their implications further in Chapter 15 and provide healthy alternatives for your baby in Chapter 16.

The 90/10 Rule

Based on the information you have read in this chapter, food items that I do not recommend as being a part of your whole pregnancy are listed below. Of course, we all have our cheat meals when there is a craving we can't possibly combat (I have been there myself!), so I ask that you commit yourself to the *The Whole Food Pregnancy Plan* 90/10 rule. Ninety percent of your food consumption will align with *The Whole Food Pregnancy Plan* philosophy, only allowing cheat items to be included in ten percent of your food intake. For example, if you eat 2,000 calories per day, ten percent of those calories can be allocated to cheat foods, which would be

---

9   JM Bell and PK Lundberg, "Effects of a commercial soy lecithin preparation on development of sensorimotor behavior and brain biochemistry in the rat.," NCBI, January 1985, accessed September 10, 2017, https://www.ncbi.nlm.nih.gov/pubmed/4038491.

90/10 Rule Gluten-Free Cheat Foods	90/10 Rule Gluten-Containing Cheat Foods
Gluten-free ice cream	Some brands of ice cream
Gluten-free candy bars	Some brands of candy bars
Gluten-free fruity candies	Some candies
Potato Chips	Some brands of chips
Kettle Corn	Cookies
Corn Chips	Bread/baked goods
Frozen Yogurt	Pancakes/waffles/French toast
Sugary Beverages	Pizza
Gluten-free cookies	Crackers
Gluten-free bread/baked goods	Fried Foods
Gluten-free pancakes/waffles/French toast	Frozen Meals
Gluten-free pizza crust	Pasta
Gluten-free crackers/cereals	Granola bars
Gluten-free fried foods	Cereal
Gluten-free frozen meals	
Gluten-free pasta	
Gluten-free granola bars	

200 calories. Cheat calories are optional and provide some wiggle room—if you choose not to take them, then more power to you! Depending on whether you live a strictly gluten-free life or not, you may also opt to delve into gluten-containing items since you can allocate your cheat calories however you choose. For those who suffer from celiac disease or just feel healthier when avoiding gluten, this list is categorized by non-gluten and gluten-containing cheat items.

The gluten-free products in the chart above are now available on the market—everything from pasta to bread to pancakes and cookies, so you may be wondering why we must restrict these items to 10 percent of our daily caloric intake since they follow the rule of being gluten-free. The food industry has capitalized on the growing number of people who are adopting a gluten-free lifestyle. If you walk down the grocery aisles, you will be inundated with gluten-free versions of almost all gluten-containing processed foods. The big misconception is that if you eat these foods then you will be healthier because you are not eating gluten. Processed foods that are labeled as gluten-free use other ingredients such as tapioca starch that will raise your blood sugar just as much (if not more) than their gluten-containing counterparts and they include the same harmful additives and preservatives. Since the above-mentioned gluten-free foods are highly processed and high-glycemic, and they are not whole food sources, they do not adhere to *The Whole Food Pregnancy Plan* principles and are not recommended; however, you can find them in the 90/10 rule cheat foods category.

Enough about the foods you shouldn't be consuming during your whole pregnancy—let's talk about all of the delicious foods you will have to choose from! You will be surprised that there is a wide variety of nutritious foods that are aligned with *The Whole Food Pregnancy Plan* philosophy and principles. The next chapter will provide your go-to grocery list which presents all of the delicious, healthy fare you will have to select from.

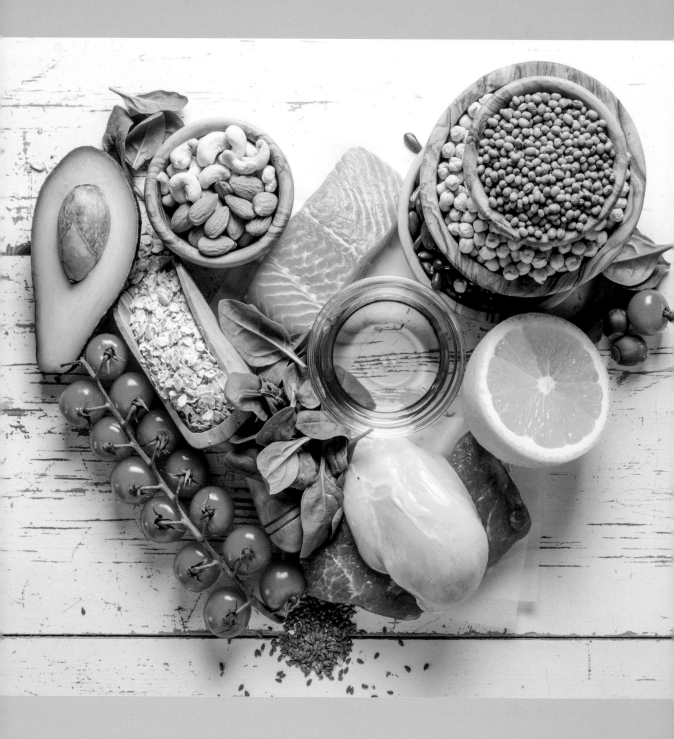

Chapter 3
The Whole Food Pregnancy Definite Dozen

I will get into specific nutrition needs based on each trimester of pregnancy in the following chapters, but if you are pregnant or trying to become pregnant, you can start stocking up on the "Definite Dozen" now as they will be used for preconception, pregnancy, postpartum weight loss, and nursing (if you choose to nurse). This chapter will provide you with an extensive grocery list; however, the following twelve food categories are vital pillars of your food regimen so please make an effort to incorporate as many of these as possible into your daily food intake. If you are a vegetarian or vegan, you will still find that over 75 percent of this "Definite Dozen" list will be suitable for your lifestyle. Both vegans and non-vegans will find many more food options in the extensive grocery list that follows.

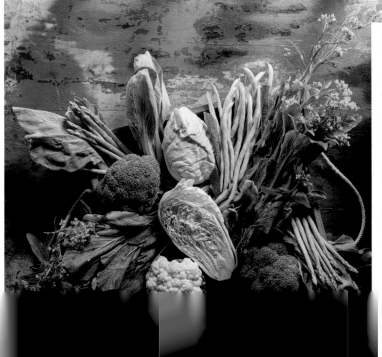

Nutrient-Dense Vegetables

It is recommended that nutrient-dense vegetables (some examples are kale, broccoli, asparagus, collard greens, cauliflower, spinach, and Brussels sprouts) make up the foundation of the prenatal diet. Eating several servings of them per day is extremely advantageous for the pregnant woman and baby. Nutrient-dense vegetables are low-sugar, unprocessed carbohydrate sources, packed with micronutrients such as folate, iron, vitamin C, and potassium, and chockful of fiber which will aid in digestion and regular bowel movements.

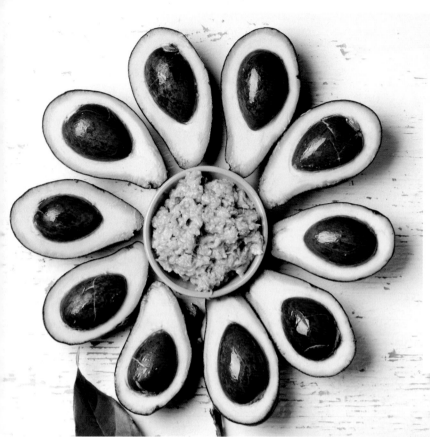

Avocado

Avocados have special properties as they are one of the only fatty fruit! Like nutrient-dense vegetables, avocados provide a variety of essential micronutrients (vitamins and minerals) as well as fiber. Avocados are a wonderful source of healthy monounsaturated fat which is critical for the development of your baby's nervous system, heart, brain, and eyes. Not to mention, good fat helps to keep you fuller for longer, fending off pesky pregnancy cravings.

Eggs

Eggs are a nice mix of quality protein and omega-3 fatty acids; protein and fat are two of the primary building blocks for fetal growth, and animal sources of omega-3 fatty acids are particularly helpful to your baby's brain and eye development. Eggs also contain choline; studies are now suggesting that choline, like folate, is critical for proper spinal cord development and adequate amounts of choline can assist in the prevention of spina bifida.

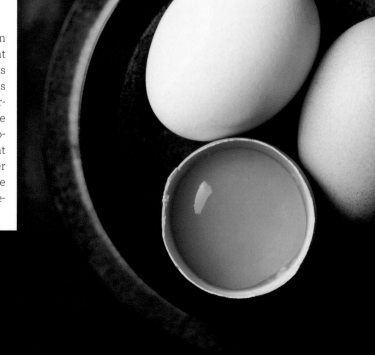

Wild Alaskan or Sockeye Salmon

In addition to being a source of protein, wild salmon (if you choose canned salmon, look for "wild Alaskan" on the label) contains omega-3 fatty acids as well. The omega-3 fats found in these types of salmon contain exceptional amounts of the vital DHA and EPA which are the long-chain omega-3s known for being most beneficial for eye, brain, and heart health.[10] In addition to their omega-3 fats, wild salmon contain high amounts of vitamin D which can be difficult to find in most foods. We will go into more detail about vitamin D in the next chapter as it is one of the most imperative nutrients for a pregnant woman to consume and the majority of us are deficient in it!

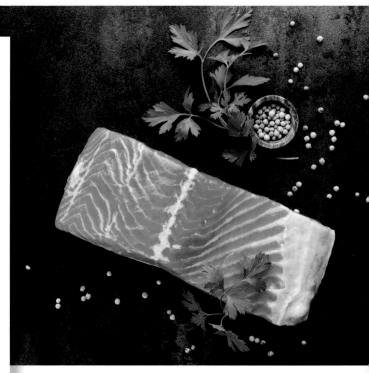

---

10 M. Singh, "Essential fatty acids, DHA and human brain.," NCBI, March 01, 2005, accessed September 05, 2017, https://www.ncbi.nlm.nih.gov/pubmed/15812120.

Low Sugar Fruits

Low sugar fruits such as tomato, bell pepper, blueberries, raspberries, and grapefruit are excellent sources of vitamin C! When you're expecting, your immune system is slightly compromised so you may be more susceptible to colds and flu and it is important to get your vitamin C but not consume too much sugar (like from orange juice) while doing so. Also a great source of fiber, these low-sugar fruits provide phytonutrients which help to prevent disease and aid in your overall well-being.

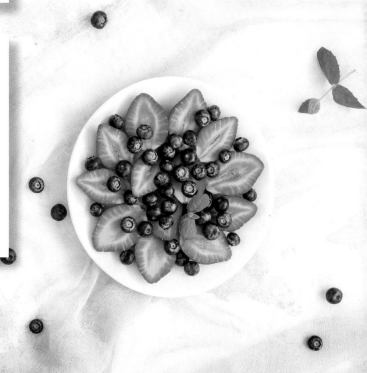

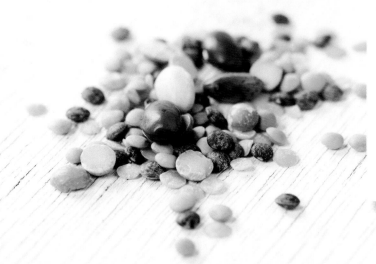

Lentils, Peas, and Beans

Lentils, peas, and beans are vegan sources of protein and iron. They also contain folate which has proven to prevent neural tube defects which are birth defects of the spine, spinal cord, and brain. In addition to protein, iron, and folate, these legumes contain a wide variety of micronutrients including but not limited to zinc, potassium, copper, and Pantothenic acid.

Sweet Potato

An excellent unprocessed, fibrous carbohydrate source, sweet potatoes will help to keep you satiated while maintaining even blood sugar levels when eaten in conjunction with extremely low-glycemic carbohydrates such as dark leafy greens. Their rich color is due to the fact that they contain the powerful antioxidant beta-carotene, which boosts your immune system and helps to fight off disease. Beta-carotene converts to vitamin A, which is necessary for mother and baby; vitamin A is important to the development of your baby's lungs, heart, kidneys, bones, and eyes, as well as the central nervous system.

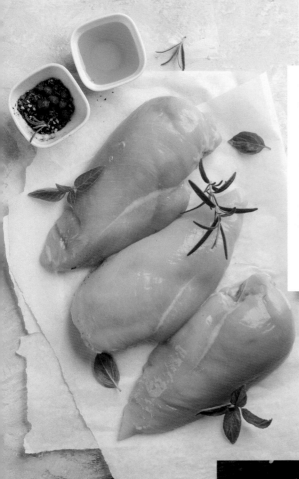

Grass-Fed, Organic Red Meat, and Organic Poultry

Due to environmental toxins found in many animal proteins, it is important to consume organic and/or grass-fed selections if possible (if you are one who consumes meat and poultry). Grass-fed red meats such as beef, lamb, and venison have high amounts of essential omega-3 fatty acids that contain DHA and EPA (like in wild salmon) in addition to their protein content. Poultry such as organic turkey and chicken provide B vitamins, iron, zinc, potassium, and phosphorus.

Nuts and Seeds

Vegan sources of protein, nuts, and seeds are packed with nutrition, providing substantial amounts of good fats, complex carbohydrates, fiber, vitamins, and minerals. Aim to consume a variety of raw nuts and seeds such as almonds, cashews, pistachios, pine nuts, walnuts, Chia seeds, and ground flaxseed to benefit from a broad spectrum of micronutrients. High in calories, a small handful as a snack or used as a topping on a salad will do!

Probiotic Foods

We all have "good" and "bad" bacteria in our bodies. Probiotics are known as the "friendly bacteria" and consist of *Lactobacillus acidophilus*, *Lactobacillus bulgarius*, *Lactobacillus reuteri*, *Streptococcus thermophiles*, *Saccharomyces boulardii*, *Bifidobacterium bifidum*, and *Bacillus subtilis*. During pregnancy, the bad bacteria tend to increase so consumption of good bacteria via probiotics may be beneficial for both mother and baby.[11] Foods that naturally contain probiotics are Greek yogurt, kefir, dairy-free kefir, apple cider vinegar, fermented soy such as tempeh and Natto (much different than unfermented soy such as tofu), and brine-cured olives. Known as a superior probiotic food, sauerkraut actually does not contain a substantially diverse amount of friendly bacteria; however, its organic acid content supports the growth of good bacteria.

11   LF Gomez Arango et al., "Probiotics and pregnancy," NCBI, January 02, 2015, accessed September 05, 2017, https://www.ncbi.nlm.nih.gov/pubmed/25398206.

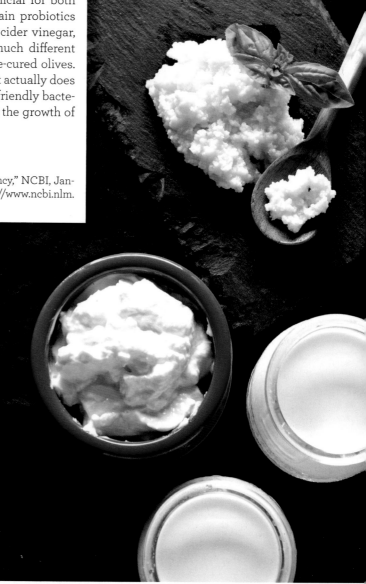

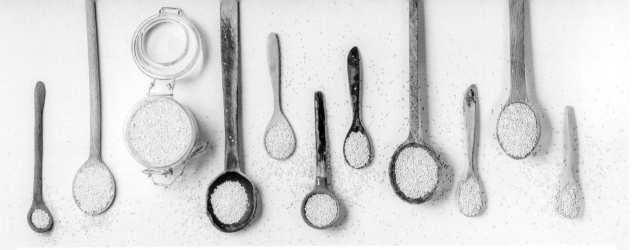

Quinoa

Sometimes mistaken for a grain, quinoa is actually classified as a seed. It contains more (and higher quality) protein than most grains and unlike most plant foods, it has all of the essential amino acids which are the building blocks of protein. This carbohydrate source will give you energy while helping to maintain even blood sugar levels.

Water

Although it's not a food, water does get a spot on the "Definite Dozen" as its importance is undeniable. Since your blood volume will increase by almost 50 percent during pregnancy, it is ideal to make a goal to drink 80 ounces of water per day. Your increased blood volume will help to transport nutrients and export wastes to and from your growing baby.

The "Definite Dozen" will lay a strong nutritional foundation to your diet and will provide much of the macro- and micro-nutrients you will need during preconception and pregnancy. I don't expect you to stick solely to the foods found in the above twelve categories, so below you will find your *Whole Food Pregnancy Plan* grocery list. If you aren't familiar with some of the items, the recipe chapters found in Chapters 18, 19, 20, and 21 will assist you with incorporating many of these foods into a variety of meals and snacks!

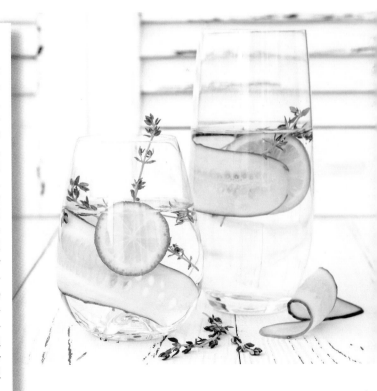

Produce		Animal Proteins	Vegan Proteins	Probiotics	Cooking Extras
☐ Apples	☐ Lemons	☐ Bison	☐ Almonds	☐ Cheddar Cheese	☐ Almond Milk
☐ Apricots	☐ Lettuce	☐ Canned Salmon	☐ Amaranth	☐ Dark Chocolate	☐ Avocado Oil
☐ Artichokes	☐ Melons	☐ Chicken	☐ Artichokes	☐ Gouda Cheese	☐ Basil
☐ Arugula	☐ Mushrooms	☐ Chunk Light Tuna	☐ Asparagus	☐ Greek Yogurt	☐ Black Pepper
☐ Asparagus	☐ Olives	☐ Clams	☐ Beans	☐ Green Olives	☐ Butter
☐ Avocados	☐ Onions	☐ Cod	☐ Black Eyed Peas	☐ Kefir	☐ Cilantro
☐ Bananas	☐ Oranges	☐ Crab	☐ Broccoli	☐ Kimchi	☐ Cinnamon
☐ Blackberries	☐ Papaya	☐ Eggs	☐ Cashews	☐ Miso (organic)	☐ Coconut Milk
☐ Blueberries	☐ Peaches	☐ Grassfed Beef	☐ Chia Seeds	☐ Mozzarella Cheese	☐ Coconut Oil
☐ Bok Choy	☐ Pears	☐ Halibut	☐ Flax Seeds	☐ Natto (organic)	☐ Extra Virgin Olive Oil
☐ Broccoli	☐ Peppers	☐ Lamb	☐ Hemp Milk	☐ Parmesan Cheese	☐ Flaxseed Oil
☐ Brussels Sprouts	☐ Plums	☐ Mussels	☐ Hemp Seeds	☐ Peas	☐ Garlic
☐ Cabbage	☐ Pomegranates	☐ Octopus	☐ Hummus	☐ Pickles	☐ Ginger
☐ Carrots	☐ Potatoes	☐ Pork	☐ Lentils	☐ Sauerkraut	☐ Gluten-Free Brewer's Yeast
☐ Cauliflower	☐ Pumpkins	☐ Rockfish	☐ Natto (organic)	☐ Swiss Cheese	☐ Grapeseed Oil
☐ Celery	☐ Raspberries	☐ Scallops	☐ Oatmeal (gluten-free)	☐ Tempeh (organic)	☐ Oregano
☐ Chard	☐ Rhubarb	☐ Shrimp	☐ Peas		☐ Paleo Mayonnaise
☐ Collard Greens	☐ Spinach	☐ Sole	☐ Pistachios		☐ Parsley
☐ Cucumbers	☐ Sprouts	☐ Squid	☐ Pumpkin Seeds		☐ Rosemary
☐ Eggplant	☐ Squash	☐ Turkey	☐ Quinoa		☐ Sage
☐ Endive	☐ Strawberries	☐ Venison	☐ Sesame Seeds		☐ Sea Salt
☐ Fennel	☐ Sweet Potatoes	☐ Wild Salmon	☐ Spinach		☐ Tahini
☐ Figs	☐ Tomatoes		☐ Spirulina		☐ Tamari
☐ Grapefruits	☐ Watermelons		☐ Tahini		☐ Tarragon
☐ Kale	☐ Zucchini		☐ Tempeh (organic)		☐ Thyme
☐ Kiwis			☐ Walnuts		☐ Turmeric

You may be wondering if you need to purchase all of the above items in order to have a successful Whole Food Pregnancy and the answer is no! The wide variety of foods found in the grocery list gives you flexibility with regard to your food lifestyle, possible allergies, and aversions. Feel free to pick and choose the groceries you prefer the most!

Chapter 4
Vitamins, Minerals & Supplements

Back in Chapter 2, I mentioned that we will be focusing on real food as opposed to synthetic vitamins—which is true! The topic of prenatal vitamins can be controversial so I am going to share my personal experience with prenatal vitamins as well as the research I conducted as a result of my experience with them. It is always best to make decisions that are suited for you, so hopefully this chapter will provide you with some information that will make your decision of whether to take prenatal vitamins or not a little bit easier. Of course, if you are someone who suffers from a severe deficiency that has been medically diagnosed by your doctor and your doctor recommends a synthetic vitamin regimen, then please follow your doctor's orders.

As you may already know, folate (or synthetic folic acid) is one of the most highly regarded prenatal nutrients as research shows that neural tube defects are reduced by 70 percent when adequate folate or folic acid has been consumed. While folate and folic acid are promoted interchangeably, their implications can be extremely different. The naturally occurring form of B9, folate is bioavailable so it absorbs more efficiently and is found in a variety of foods. Folic acid is the synthetic form of folate and is largely found in fortified foods and supplements. Not only do our bodies use folate more efficiently, we are also adept at regulating folate levels in our bloodstream as it is capable of being excreted through urine. Synthetic folic acid does not metabolize in the same manner and one must closely regulate how much synthetic folic acid is consumed as too much can lead to toxicity.[12]

It is recommended by the American Pregnancy Association that pregnant women consume 400–800 micrograms of folate or synthetic folic acid every day. There are a variety of ways in which you

---

12 F. Scaglione and G. Panzavolta, "Folate, folic acid and 5-methyltetrahydrofolate are not the same thing," NCBI, May 2014, accessed September 05, 2017, https://www.ncbi.nlm.nih.gov/pubmed/24494987.

can obtain naturally occurring folate as it can be found in many foods. I will give several examples of folate foods in later chapters but for now, here is an example of a combination of four simple foods that will provide you with 600 micrograms of folate:

¾ cup of lentils: 268 micrograms
1 cup of boiled asparagus: 262 micrograms
½ cup of avocado: 55 micrograms
½ cup of strawberries: 20 micrograms

Since 600 micrograms of folic acid can be easy to find in prenatal vitamins as opposed to preparing foods like the ones mentioned above, you may be wondering why I am discussing the possibility of not taking prenatal vitamins since it is mainstream consensus that supplement intake is standard protocol for prenatal health. In reality, obtaining nutrients from real food as opposed to synthetic vitamins is ideal for the human body, especially the pregnant human body. If one truly has a poor diet and is not willing to make any adjustments then yes, a prenatal vitamin may be imperative, but if one consumes folate-rich foods like the selections above then the folic acid in a prenatal vitamin may be unnecessary.

I found out I was pregnant on December 11, 2014, and my doctor estimated that we conceived around November 10, 2014. She asked me if I had been taking any prenatal vitamins and my reply was that I had not since I didn't even realize I was pregnant. The doctor urged that I drive directly from her office to a store where I could buy some prenatal vitamins since I would be in desperate need of folic acid to prevent neural tube defects such as spina bifida. In a mild panic, I obliged and distinctly remember darting straight to the store, ripping open the package, and taking the vitamin while still standing in the pill aisle. What I was not aware of at the time is that spina bifida occurs within three to four weeks after conception; when I started my prenatal vitamin regimen, I was already in week five of pregnancy! Thankfully, my pre-pregnancy diet included a steady routine of high-folate foods such as Brussels sprouts and lentils, so my personal need for folic acid supplementation through a multi-vitamin happened to be unnecessary.

I continued to take my prenatal vitamins for the other nutrients they contain and soon became constipated on a very regular basis. I had heard about pregnancy constipation so I just assumed it was a normal change my body was going through and that I would just have to deal with it. Coincidentally, it was at this time that I really started to research my prenatal vitamins as I was curious about exactly what I was putting into my body every day since I'm not normally one who takes vitamins or medications. After learning about the implications of synthetic folic acid versus naturally occurring folate, I began to wonder how the synthetic forms of other nutrients found in the pills may be affecting me.

Pregnant women need twenty-seven milligrams of iron every day; ferrous sulfate is a mineral that supplies iron to your body and it is commonly found in prenatal vitamins. What I was not aware of at the time is that ferrous sulfate is one of the leading iron supplements that is known for causing constipation, nausea, and other gastrointestinal issues.[13] Constipation and nausea are present for many pregnant women, solely due to the changes that our bodies experience when expecting. Compounding these issues with a supplement that promotes even more constipation and nausea is counterintuitive but possibly something to explore if it means that exceptional iron stores are given in exchange. When taken on an empty stomach, the effects of ferrous sulfate on the stomach can be more likely and unfortunately, the absorption rate of ferrous sulfate when taken with food is cut down by two-thirds. Iron from animal sources (meat, fish, poultry, eggs) have an absorption rate of 15–35 percent and the ability for the iron to absorb is less affected by extenuating circumstances.[14]

> Iron levels are routinely checked during pregnancy, so it will be relatively easy for your healthcare practitioner to determine whether you are meeting your body's iron needs through diet alone or if supplements are truly necessary.[15]
> **—Katie Williams, RN, BSN, PHN**

---

13   Z. Tolkien, L. Stecher, and J. Powell, "Ferrous Sulfate Supplementation Causes Significant Gastrointestinal Side-Effects in Adults: A Systematic Review and Meta-Analysis," NCBI, February 20, 2015, accessed September 06, 2017, https://www.ncbi.nlm.nih.gov/pmc/articles/PMC4336293/pdf/pone.0117383.pdf.

14   N. Abbaspour, R. Hurrell, and R. Kelishadi, "Review on iron and its importance for human health," NCBI, November 27, 2013, accessed September 06, 2017, https://www.ncbi.nlm.nih.gov/pmc/articles/PMC3999603/#__ffn_sectitle.

15   The American Congress of Obstetricians and Gynecologists: https://www.acog.org/Patients/FAQs/Routine-Tests-During-Pregnancy

I went on to explore the calcium carbonate found in my prenatal vitamins which is a calcium supplement made from chalk, limestone, and the shells of shellfish. Pregnant women do need sufficient calcium as it will assist with your baby's teeth and bone development; if one does not get proper calcium intake, the baby will draw calcium directly from the mother's body via her bones. Calcium can be found in natural food sources such as sunflower seeds, green beans, clams, figs, broccoli, sweet potatoes, oranges, almonds, and butternut squash.

Some studies have shown that calcium carbonate found in prenatal vitamins can actually reduce bone mineral content in some women.[16] In addition, calcium carbonate interferes with the absorption of the ferrous sulfate (mineral that supplies iron) when taken together, and they are automatically taken together since prenatal vitamins contain them in one pill.[17] Another fact to consider is that calcium carbonate is known to contain lead. Of course they contain trace amounts of lead that are still deemed acceptable by the FDA but one must ponder the risks and rewards of calcium carbonate consumption when all of the facts are presented.

My prenatal vitamins also contained vitamin D and yes, vitamin D is one of the most critical micronutrients for pregnant women. Not all vitamin D is considered equal—there is vitamin D2 and vitamin D3, and they are not interchangeable. Several brands of prenatal vitamins (including the ones I took) contain vitamin D2, however vitamin D3 is more powerful and effective.[19] In addition, there is a fine line between an effective dose of vitamin D2 and toxicity.

As mentioned before, your choice to take prenatal vitamins is a personal one and should be based on your unique situation. I cannot recommend or discourage prenatal vitamins as they may be needed by some but not for

16   L. MA Jarjou et al., "Unexpected long-term effects of calcium supplementation in pregnancy on maternal bone outcomes in women with a low calcium intake: a follow-up study1,2,3," NCBI, June 13, 2013, accessed September 06, 2017, https://www.ncbi.nlm.nih.gov/pmc/articles/PMC3743734/.

17   PA Seligman et al., "Measurements of iron absorption from prenatal multivitamin--mineral supplements.," NCBI, March 1983, accessed September 05, 2017, https://www.ncbi.nlm.nih.gov/pubmed/6823378.

18   Heringhausen, J., & Montgomery, K. S. (2005). Continuing Education Module—Maternal Calcium Intake and Metabolism During Pregnancy and Lactation. *The Journal of Perinatal Education*, 14(1), 52–57. http://doi.org/10.1624/105812405X23621

19   L. Tripkovic et al., "Comparison of vitamin D2 and vitamin D3 supplementation in raising serum 25-hydroxyvitamin D status: a systematic review and meta-analysis1,2,3," NCBI, May 02, 2012, accessed September 05, 2017, https://www.ncbi.nlm.nih.gov/pmc/articles/PMC3349454/#!po=78.1250.

While maternal stores of calcium are transferred readily to the growing fetus, the mother's body has been shown to physiologically adapt to this increased need for calcium without the need for increased dietary calcium or supplements. This occurs through special interactions between a parathyroid hormone, calcitonin, and vitamin D. In other words, the mother's body not only produces more calcium during pregnancy, it absorbs it more readily and uses it more efficiently. Maternal calcium levels will return to normal at the cessation of pregnancy or breastfeeding without the use of supplements. Studies have shown, however, that calcium supplements can help prevent pregnancy-induced hypertension (PIH) and preeclampsia, so it is important to discuss all options with your doctor or midwife in order to make a medically-safe, informed decision.[18]

—Katie Williams, RN, BSN, PHN

others, depending on individual nutrition regimens. Even though I took prenatal vitamins during half of my pregnancy, if I become pregnant again, I will opt to only focus on nutrient-dense foods with zero synthetic vitamin supplementation. Hopefully, the details I presented above will help you with your decision as well!

There are three supplements that I definitely find beneficial while you are expecting (or trying to conceive). Probiotics, krill oil, and vitamin D3 are advantageous to anyone's diet but can be especially valuable for an expectant mother and fetus. Just like with prenatal vitamins, I will present some details about probiotics, krill oil, and vitamin D3 to help

you with your research. As always, be sure to consult your doctor if you have questions or concerns.

Probiotics

Our bodies contain good and bad bacteria; probiotics are known as the "friendly" bacteria as they help to neutralize bad bacteria. Three of the most regularly consumed probiotics include *Lactobacillus*, *Bifidobacterium*, and *Saccharomyces*. They can be found in pill form, Greek yogurt, and a variety of fermented foods. Studies have suggested that probiotics assist with the prevention of preterm labor, gestational diabetes, bladder infections, ear infections, bacterial vaginosis, inflammatory bowel disease, and some allergies.[20] It is common that as a woman's pregnancy progresses, so does the incidence of bad bacteria, so offsetting the bad bacteria with "friendly" bacteria found in probiotics may be favorable. According to the National Library of Medicine and the National Institute of Health, there is little risk in taking probiotics during pregnancy or while nursing.

Omega-3 Fatty Acids

Throughout this book, I recommend several food sources of omega-3 fatty acids, however, if you feel as if you are not eating enough of those good fats, you may want to consider supplementing. While we do require omega-6 fatty acids, studies have shown that the majority of pregnant women have an overabundance of omega-6 (these are prevalent in inferior oils, processed foods, and fast food) and not enough omega-3 (these are prevalent in foods such as fish, eggs, seaweed, walnuts). While consuming plant-based omega-3 fatty acids is beneficial, the most superior source of omega-3 fatty

acids come from animal products such as wild salmon, as those omega-3s contain DHA (docosahexaenoic acid) which is the omega-3 that plays the most critical role in fetal brain and eye development. If you are a vegan or vegetarian, one of the best sources of DHA is seaweed. Most other plant-based omega-3s contain ALA (alpha-linolenic acid) which converts into a minimal amount of DHA. [21]

I do recommend animal-sourced omega-3 fatty acid supplementation if you do not get this fat from your food intake since your baby will need to acquire DHA from the placenta to assist with fetal brain and eye development. Fish oil is an option (I prefer wild Alaskan salmon oil due to less environmental toxins). Another source of DHA with even fewer environmental toxins is krill oil—krill are little crustaceans that feed on phytoplankton and are harvested in the Antarctic. Krill oil was my most consumed omega-3 supplement during my own pregnancy, but please feel free to do further research to see if it is right for you!

---

20   LF Gomez Arango et al., "Probiotics and pregnancy," NCBI, January 2015, accessed September 10, 2017, https://www.ncbi.nlm.nih.gov/pubmed/25398206.

21   J. Coletta, S. Bell, and A. Roman, "Omega-3 Fatty Acids and Pregnancy," NCBI, October 2010, accessed September 10, 2017, https://www.ncbi.nlm.nih.gov/pmc/articles/PMC3046737/.

Vitamin D3

A large majority of our population is deficient in vitamin D and this can be disadvantageous during pregnancy. Although more research is needed, some studies have shown associations of maternal vitamin D deficiency with preterm birth, low birth weight, preecamplsia and gestational diabetes.[22] In addition, since vitamin D is needed to maintain sufficient levels of calcium and phosphorus, a lack of vitamin D during pregnancy can result in abnormal fetal bone growth and fractures.[23] The amount of vitamin D a pregnant women should supplement with is up for debate by many medical associations and recommendations range from 600 International Units (IU) to 4,000 International Units. According to the American Pregnancy Association, there was a recent study that concluded that daily consumption of 4,000 International Units (IU) of vitamin D by expecting women had the most benefit with regard to preventing premature labors (and births), as well as infections. In addition, the study reported the consumption of 4,000 IU on a daily basis to be harmless to mother and baby.[24] Some establishments recommend a lower dose so please consult your doctor regarding this matter to find out what is best for you.

One fact that is likely is that if you are depending on a prenatal vitamin

Vitamin D is not only beneficial in aiding calcium absorption, it helps regulate your circadian rhythm as well! If your newborn has day/night reversal, make sure she gets a good dose of indirect sunlight, especially in the morning. Just fifteen minutes a day can help her body adjust, and will likely eliminate those long nighttime awake periods within a week or two.[25]

—Katie Williams, RN, BSN, PHN

22 R. Urrutia and J. Thorp, "Vitamin D in Pregnancy: Current Concepts," NCBI, March 2012, accessed September 11, 2017, https://www.ncbi.nlm.nih.gov/pmc/articles/PMC3709246/.

23 P. Mahon et al., "Low maternal vitamin D status and fetal bone development: cohort study," NCBI, January 2010, accessed September 11, 2017, https://www.ncbi.nlm.nih.gov/pmc/articles/PMC4768344/.

24 S. Al Emadi and M. Hammoudeh, "Vitamin D study in pregnant women and their babies," NCBI, November 01, 2013, accessed September 11, 2017, https://www.ncbi.nlm.nih.gov/pmc/articles/PMC3991049/.

25 McGraw K, Hoffmann R, Harker C, Herman JH. (1999 May). The Development of Circadian Rhythms in a Human Infant. *Sleep*, 1;22(3):303–10.

for sufficient vitamin D levels, the 400 International Units (IU) found in most prenatal vitamins probably isn't enough. Also, as I mentioned earlier in this chapter, many prenatal vitamins contain vitamin D2 and that does not absorb well; vitamin D3 is far superior. Vitamin D is only available in a few foods (see table below) so it is very difficult to get sufficient vitamin D from food alone. If you live in an area where it is possible, responsible sun exposure will do wonders for vitamin D levels. Direct sunlight on as much of your body's surface as possible for around 10–15 minutes per day (with no sunscreen and not through a window) is very substantial. If this is not possible during a certain time of year, you may want to consider taking vitamin D3 supplements or fish oil.

As you can see, it is very difficult to reach optimal vitamin D levels without supplementing or receiving responsible

Source of Vitamin D	International Units (IU) Per Serving
Fish Oil	1,000
Sockeye Salmon (3 ounces)	447
Canned Tuna (3 ounces)	154
Some brands of yogurt (6 ounces)	80
Sardines (two whole sardines)	46
Beef liver, cooked (3 ounces)*	42
Whole egg (1 large)	41
Swiss cheese (1 ounce)	6

*Some studies suggest the benefits of consuming liver during pregnancy outweigh risks.[26]

sun exposure. Adding these vitamin D sources into your daily food regimen will assist with your levels, however, you may want to consult with your doctor about taking vitamin D3 in pill form. You can find all of the above mentioned supplements (probiotics, krill oil, fish oil, vitamin D3) at a variety of grocery, vitamin, and health stores.

---

26   Michael Nelson, "Vitamin A, liver consumption, and risk of birth defects," NCBI, November 24, 1990, accessed October 01, 2017, https://www.ncbi.nlm.nih.gov/pmc/articles/PMC1664333/pdf/bmj00207-0012.pdf.

Chapter 5
Pregnancy Nutrition Myths

I got so many questions while I was pregnant—primarily about the different foods I was and was *not* eating. Some of my responses drew looks of concern and even more resulted in genuine surprise and confusion. The myths I'm about to go over stem from general blanket statements that have little to no credible statistics or research to back them up. Unfortunately, these myths—some of which are primary culprits in the deteriorating health of pregnant women—have spread throughout society as being legitimate and thus are followed by the masses.

Myth ① You need whole wheat bread, pasta, and cereal to get your fiber!

Excellent marketing by the food industry has made people believe these items are good sources of fiber. The truth is that you can get much more fiber per calorie in other sources of non-processed, natural foods. Below I compare different food sources of fiber, and how much one must eat to obtain thirty grams of fiber.

FOOD	Calories Consumed to Reach 30 Grams of Fiber	Carbohydrates Consumed to Reach 30 Grams of Fiber	Sodium Consumed to Reach 30 Grams of Fiber
Whole Wheat Bread	1,350	270g	2025mg
Multi-Grain Cereal	1,275	275g	2300mg
Whole Wheat Pasta	1,260	246g	20mg
Flaxseed	550	30g	30mg
Pear with Skin	515	140g	10mg
Split Peas	495	90g	15mg
Lentils	480	90g	15mg
Broccoli	465	90g	450mg
Chia Seeds	385	33g	13mg
Raspberries	240	56g	4mg
Artichoke Hearts	195	45g	200mg

In addition to having more fiber per calorie, natural foods such as broccoli, raspberries, artichoke hearts, pears, flaxseed, Chia seeds, split peas, and lentils are non-processed and contain no artificial additives, but most commercially-made breads, pastas, and cereals do. Whole foods are superior when it comes to vitamins and minerals too. Breads and cereals are fortified with vitamins, which means they do not occur naturally and therefore, they are harder to absorb. The next time you are in a grocery store, look at the ingredient labels of breads, pastas, and cereals— you'll find a plethora of ingredients (such as sugar, high fructose corn syrup, and preservatives) that are not ideal for the growing fetus or the mother.

Myth ② You need several servings of whole wheat bread, pasta, and cereal to get your carbs!

Many pregnancy nutrition resources recommend as much as 300 grams (or sometimes more) of carbohydrates per day for an expectant mother, most of which come from gluten-containing foods such as whole wheat bread, pasta, and cereal. These types of carbohydrates are high-glycemic which means they turn into a lot of sugar! Over-consumption of sugar is one of the primary causes of gestational diabetes and the sugar you don't burn off turns to fat, so it is critical to keep sugars and high-glycemic carbohydrates to a minimum. The best sources of carbohydrates are low-glycemic, meaning they don't raise your blood sugar levels. Low-glycemic examples of carbohydrates are green vegetables, berries, grapefruit, avocado, quinoa, beans, lentils, Greek yogurt, and almonds. Not only do these items contain carbohydrates that can be used for energy, they are non- or minimally-processed and have an abundance of naturally occurring nutrients.

Myth ③ Don't eat fish!

Yes, there are some fish to avoid if pregnant due to high mercury content such as tilefish, shark, swordfish, and mackerel. On the other hand, there are many types of fish that are extremely beneficial to the mother and growing baby. Wild salmon, for example, is relatively low in mercury but high in protein and omega-3 fatty acids. As discussed previously, omega-3 fatty acids are crucial for fetal brain and retina development. I personally ate two to three servings of low-mercury fish per week while I was pregnant. According to the Natural Resources Defense Council, the following listed sea foods are the lowest in mercury.

Anchovies, Butterfish, Catfish, Clam, Crab (Domestic), Crawfish/Crayfish, Croaker (Atlantic), Flounder, Haddock (Atlantic), Hake, Herring, Mullet, Oyster, Perch (Ocean), Plaice, Pollock, Salmon (Canned), Salmon (Fresh), Sardine, Scallop, Shad (American), Shrimp, Sole (Pacific), Squid (Calamari), Trout (Freshwater), and Whitefish.

You will see in following chapters, a few *Whole Food Pregnancy* meals and recipes include canned tuna. I recommend chunk-light tuna since it is three times lower in mercury than solid white albacore. According to the American Pregnancy Association, no more than six ounces of albacore tuna should be consumed per week.

Myth ④ Drink lots of milk to get your calcium!

Once again, the marketing for milk has been genius—it does a body good, right? Or not so much. First of all, as I mentioned earlier, cow's milk has hormones in it which help to grow very large cows! Even if you choose the organic brands, the hormones (intended for cows) still remain. Milk is touted for its calcium content and is known for building strong bones but some studies suggest that calcium found in cow's milk has no correlation with strong bones and prevention of fractures.[27] Not to mention, at twelve grams of sugar per cup, it's not the ideal beverage for a pregnant woman. For more beneficial sources of calcium, please refer to the table on the next page.

Myth ⑤ Eat for two!

During your first trimester, you do not need any extra calories—your baby is the size of a blueberry! You will need a few hundred extra calories towards the middle and end of your pregnancy but let's consider this—the average baby is around seven pounds at full gestation so even at nine months pregnant, you still

---

27 D. Feskanich et al., "Milk, dietary calcium, and bone fractures in women: a 12-year prospective study," NCBI, June 1997, accessed September 11, 2017, https://www.ncbi.nlm.nih.gov/pmc/articles/PMC1380936/.

FOOD	SERVING	CALORIES	CALCIUM (mg)	SUGAR (g)
Sardines	3.5 Ounce Can	210	351	0
Sesame Seeds	¼ Cup	206	351	0
Collard Greens (cooked)	1 Cup	49	300	1
Spinach (cooked)	1 Cup	41	245	1
Canned Salmon	4 ounces	155	232	0
White Beans	1 Cup	299	126	1
Fresh Wild Salmon	6 Ounces	300	120	0
Kale (raw)	1 Cup	33	101	0
Almonds	23 Almonds	162	75	1
Orange	1 Whole	45	74	9

will not need to "eat for two." And let's face it, pregnant women have cravings (I know I did) so most of us are probably getting those few extra hundred calories in per day, if you know what I mean! In most cases, there won't be a need to consciously add in more food to your daily routine—simply eat when you are hungry and stop when you are full.

Myth ⑥ You can eat whatever you want!

"You're pregnant! You deserve to eat whatever you want!" No!!! You are growing a human! This is *the* most important time to eat the most nourishing foods possible. Eating "whatever you want" may lead to excessive weight gain and health problems for mother and baby. Unfortunately, half of all pregnant women are overweight or obese.

Myth ⑦ You can get everything you need from prenatal vitamins!

I talked about prenatal vitamins in Chapter 4 but I am mentioning it again here as synthetic vitamin intake (as opposed to obtaining naturally occurring vitamins from food) has become a popular, quick fix among pregnant women. Prenatal vitamins are synthetic versions of real vitamins—they are made in a lab! Typical food intake of the general population lacks essential vitamins and nutrients which creates the need for the ever-expanding market of fortified nutrients. If you eat a balanced diet of whole foods, you will get what you and your growing baby need. Prenatal vitamins are not easily absorbed and contain things like folic acid and ferrous sulfate—inferior versions of folate and iron.

Myth ⑧ Stay away from fat!

It is true that many fats should be limited or avoided during pregnancy but not all fats are created equally! We tend to overdose on omega-6 fats which are found in items such as processed foods, vegetable oil, fast food, cookies, chips, and French fries, and then lack the omega-3 fats that are most beneficial during pregnancy. omega-3 fats are found in foods such as wild salmon, walnuts, flaxseed, and grass-fed meats. These fats are not only beneficial to the mother but they also play a key role in fetal brain/eye development and is beneficial for maternal heart health.

Myth ⑨ Keep hydrated with Gatorade and juices!

Fluid needs increase dramatically during pregnancy due to your increasing blood volume but this doesn't mean that it's beneficial to load up on beverages such as sports drinks, fruit juices, or vitamin water. Making water your primary source of hydration while pregnant is critical. Of course, sports drinks and vitamin enhanced waters boast electrolytes and fortified (fake) nutrients but what comes along with these electrolytes and nutrients is a whole lot of sugar, artificial coloring, and preservatives. Want some ideas for homemade, natural beverages that boast electrolytes? Refer to Chapter 14!

Myth ⑩ Your pregnancy weight gain will directly reflect your baby's weight gain!

At week forty of my pregnancy (I didn't deliver until I was forty-one weeks and five days along), I had gained a total of twenty-three pounds. Throughout my pregnancy, my doctor had warned me several times that I was not gaining enough weight. After returning home from a two-week vacation to Europe when I was 7.5 months pregnant, she exclaimed, "Who doesn't gain weight while on vacation?! Go home and eat some ice cream." At a check-up in my ninth month of pregnancy, my doctor said that based on my weight gain, the baby would be "around six pounds but no more than 6.5 pounds." Although my weight gain was "low" for American standards, my diet was crammed full with quality proteins and good fats, along with a moderate amount of low-glycemic carbohydrates. When my son was born, he was put on my chest for skin-to-skin contact in order to initiate breast-feeding before he was weighed and got his APGAR scores. I could tell that he was big but I would still be shocked to find out that he was a whopping nine pounds and twelve ounces—just the weight of an apple short of ten pounds!

My doctor warned that my "low" weight gain would result in a small baby but clearly, the opposite can happen as well. There are unfortunate and scary scenarios in which pregnant women will gain upwards of seventy pounds, get rushed in for an emergency C-section due to a "large baby," but then the baby ends up weighing five pounds. Many of these scenarios are a result of poor diet and nutrition. The growing fetus thrives on proper nutrition, including quality proteins and healthy fats. If one's diet is rich in junk food, processed foods, and sugar, and devoid of essential nutrients, it is possible that the fetus will not develop and grow at an ideal rate. The excess sugar and carbohydrates get stored on the mother causing her to gain weight and the baby to lack what she needs to reach average or above average size. Of course, the opposite can happen as well—excessive maternal weight gain can also lead to large babies who suffer from hypoglycemia which results from a maternal diet that is full of sugar and high-glycemic carbohydrates, so it is best to stick to a nutritious diet, while indulging in moderation.

You will receive a lot of advice (good and bad) when you are pregnant—hopefully, I cleared up some confusion for you by dispelling some of these popular myths. Pregnancy nutrition can be complicated due to the never-ending and conflicting resources that are available today. To avoid implementing potentially harmful nutrition practices while expecting, always do your own research and consult with your health care professional to determine what is best for you and your baby.

Chapter 6
The Importance of Pre-Pregnancy Nutrition

We have all heard the saying "You are what you eat." Once you conceive, your baby is what you eat as well. In fact, much of what you eat long before conception plays an imperative role in the development of the embryo and fetus so adequate nutrition should be a part of your daily lifestyle at least three months before you become pregnant. The first eight weeks after conception are particularly critical for the embryo to receive exceptional care and one of the biggest influences you can control is what you put in your body. Unfortunately, if you wait until you have taken a positive pregnancy test to start nourishing yourself properly, your child will not receive vital nutrients that are essential in the very early stages of conception since your body needs time to "become what it eats."

Whether you have no known fertility issues or you are having trouble with conceiving, this chapter is for you. The foods discussed here are for both providing exceptional nutrients for the embryo in the early stages of conception as well as furnishing the best foods for women who want to increase chances of fertility. Studies now correlate the typical Western diet of grains, processed foods, and sugar with raised rates of infertility.[28] These studies recommend following a "good diet," but one's idea of a "good diet" is open to interpretation especially with all of the conflicting information that can be found on the Internet, in books, or even in your doctor's office. In a nutshell, studies now suggest that carbohydrates from vegetables, sweet potatoes, squash, some fruits, and healthy fats from foods such as avocado, grass-fed meats, and eggs optimize one's fertility.[29]

---

28 P. Nazni, "Association of western diet & lifestyle with decreased fertility," NCBI, November 2014, accessed September 11, 2017, https://www.ncbi.nlm.nih.gov/pmc/articles/PMC4345758/.

29 P. Nazni, "Association of western diet & lifestyle with decreased fertility," NCBI, November 2014, accessed September 11, 2017, https://www.ncbi.nlm.nih.gov/pmc/articles/PMC4345758/.

There are several ways that having celiac disease or NCGS can affect your ability to get pregnant, stay pregnant, the overall health and development of your baby in-utero, delivery, breastfeeding, and beyond. The major factor is malnutrition related to the destruction of the villi in the small intestine (duodenum, jejunem, and ileum) preventing food from being broken down and absorbed as nutrients or fuel for your body. And this malnutrition can show up in people that are underweight, normal weight, and overweight. For some people, this can show up as deficiencies in iron, folate, B12 (pernicious anemia), fat soluble vitamins such as A, D, E, and K, zinc, calcium, and magnesium, especially magnesium in the red blood cells (rbc) or any other nutrient. Please consider that preeclampsia is emergently treated with magnesium to prevent seizures. How are these mothers getting to be deficient in magnesium, especially if they are taking prenatal vitamins? Perhaps undiagnosed celiac disease is the answer. If the mother is unable to absorb nutrients then her growing fetus is not going to have access to the necessary nutrients available for proper growth and development. It is important to identify women and their partners as celiac well before they try to become pregnant because these undiagnosed moms (and dads) will have a difficult time getting pregnant and maintaining a pregnancy for full-term. Ideally, people will allow their own bodies at least one year to heal before they actively try to get pregnant. The inflammation, intestinal organ damage, damaged immune system and deficiencies can all effectively be resolved, but it takes typically at least a year.

—Nadine Grzeskowiak, RN, BSN, CEN

Before I discuss exactly what you should be eating during this time, there are four common, erroneous pre-conception nutrition recommendations that I would like to address first as avoiding them could positively affect your ability to conceive. In addition, sidestepping these food industry–advocated suggestions from the start will help you form healthy habits that will last for the duration of your pregnancy. Common recommendations to *avoid* are:

- Consume three servings of milk/dairy (including ice cream) per day for protein, fat, calcium, and vitamin D.

- Drink 2–3 servings of processed/commercial fruit juice per day for vitamin C and calcium.
- Eat several servings of high-starch, high-carbohydrate gluten-foods such as bread, pasta, and cereal per day for folic acid, energy, and fiber.
- Consume low-fat foods.
- Use synthetic folic acid as a substitute for naturally occurring folate.

It is fact that fat, protein, energy, fiber, calcium, folate, vitamins C and D are essential for conception and embryonic health, however, the negatives of these above mentioned suggestions far outweigh the positives. These conventional recommendations should actually be avoided as they lead expecting women down a dangerous path of potential diet-related pregnancy complications including gestational diabetes, excessive weight gain, and iron-deficiency; not to mention, they could possibly prevent conception to begin with. Let's explore each one of these recommendations along with the implications of consuming these foods while trying to conceive.

Cow's Milk

The marketing of cow's milk has been quite extensive, leading the masses to believe that it is a superior beverage due to its calcium, added vitamin D, and protein. Milk is especially promoted to pregnant women and women who are trying to conceive but studies are now showing that the negatives may be outweighed by the positives of cow's milk consumption. For example, as we all know, building iron stores during pre-conception and pregnancy is essential as the fetus acquires iron from her mother. There are conflicting reports regarding the effects of casein, phosphate, and calcium (found in cow's milk) and how it inhibits iron absorption.[30] In fact, a recent study documented in the New Zealand Medical Journal reports that drinking three or more cups of milk per day during pregnancy may negatively affect brain fetal brain development due to insufficient iron stores.[31]

---

30 LS Jackson and K. Lee, "The effect of dairy products on iron availability," NCBI, September 29, 2009, accessed September 13, 2017, https://www.ncbi.nlm.nih.gov/pubmed/1581006.

31 S. Morton et al., "Maternal and perinatal predictors of newborn iron status," New Zealand Medical Journal, September 12, 2014, accessed September 13, 2017, https://www.nzma.org.nz/journal/read-the-journal/all-issues/2010–2019/2014/vol-127-no-1402/6293.

Commercial cow's milk contains hormones that are meant for cows, not humans. Even the organic brands of milk contain hormones that are naturally found in the animal. A rising concern is that modern pregnant cows continue to lactate so they, too, are used in commercial milk production. The milk that comes from pregnant cows has considerably high levels of estrogens and progesterone which are absorbed by whoever is drinking the milk. This hormone absorption is linked with earlier sexual maturation in children as well as lowered levels of testosterone in males.[32] These are some alarming factors to take into consideration when pondering the common recommendation that you should be consuming three servings of dairy per day, every day while you are expecting.

At twelve grams of sugar and thirteen grams of carbohydrates per cup of milk and twenty-one grams of sugar and twenty-nine grams of carbohydrates per half cup of ice cream, the three recommended servings (two cups of milk and a half cup ice cream) of dairy potentially leads to forty-five grams of sugar and fifty-five grams of carbohydrates per day without taking any other foods/beverages into consideration. As discussed in Chapter 1, limiting sugar intake before and during pregnancy is instrumental in avoiding gestational diabetes which affects up to 10 percent of all pregnant women in the United States. You may be thinking that twelve grams of sugar per cup of milk is worth the benefits of the calcium milk will provide you with regard to your bone health but ironically, many studies now show that milk may be associated with higher incidence of fractures.[33]

Fruit Juice

In addition to cow's milk, commercial fruit juice is a conventional beverage that is included in standard preconception diets. Fruit juices do contain some essential vitamins but those vitamins come with a cost and that cost is an overabundance of fructose (sugar from fruit). The average American consumes eighty-eight grams of sugar per day—that's equivalent to

32 K. Maruyama, T. Oshima, and K. Ohyama, "Exposure to exogenous estrogen through intake of commercial milk produced from pregnant cows." NCBI, February 2010, accessed September 20, 2017, https://www.ncbi.nlm.nih.gov/pubmed/19496976.

33 K. Michaëlsson et al., "Milk intake and risk of mortality and fractures in women and men: cohort studies." NCBI, October 28, 2014, accessed September 20, 2017, https://www.ncbi.nlm.nih.gov/pubmed/25352269.

twenty-two teaspoons! It is a common misconception that sugar from fruit juice is harmless since it comes from a natural source. Unfortunately, whether you consume sugar from a candy bar or sugar from a glass of juice, your body will have the same reaction—raised blood sugar levels followed by insulin release. Below we compare the whole fruit with its corresponding juice in terms of calories, sugar, and fiber.

	CALORIES	SUGAR	FIBER
1 Orange	45	9 g	2.3 g
Orange Juice (1 Cup)	111	21 g	0.5 g
1 Apple	78	15 g	3.6 g
Apple Juice (1 Cup)	113	24 g	0.5 g
½ Large Grapefruit	52	8 g	2 g
Grapefruit Juice (1 Cup)	96	18 g	0.2 g

As most foods that are found on shelves and in packages, the processing of juice strips some of the nutrients such as fiber that occur naturally in the whole fruit. I suggest eating the actual piece of fruit accompanied by a glass of water. This combination will hydrate and deliver fiber, calcium, potassium, and vitamin C with only a fraction of the calories and sugar found in juice.

Getting in the habit of drinking water (as opposed to milk, juice, or soda) as your primary beverage now will greatly benefit you and your baby. An expectant mother should aim to consume at least eighty ounces of water per day as it keeps you hydrated and delivers nutrients to your embryo. As you move forward with your pregnancy, your blood volume will begin to increase and the best fluid to aid in that increase is good old H2O!

Bread, Pasta, and Cereal

Most popular guidelines advise to eat several servings of these items every day for energy, fiber, and fortified folic acid. As previously mentioned, gestational diabetes is prevalent the United States and this is partially to blame on overconsumption of high-carbohydrate, high-glycemic gluten-foods including bread, pasta, cereal, and crackers. Also, if you are one of the five million women in the United States who currently suffers from Polycystic Ovary Syndrome, it is critical to limit high-glycemic carbohydrates such as these since high levels of insulin (which happens in response to high-carbohydrate consumption) can interrupt ovulation.[34] You can acquire many of your carbohydrates from low-glycemic green vegetables, lentils, beans, and low sugar fruits such as blueberries and avocado. These whole foods are unprocessed and boast a variety of naturally occurring nutrients such as folate, versus the synthetic folic acid found in highly processed, fortified breads and cereals.

Low-fat Fad

Several current medical and nutritional resources are still recommending that pregnant women (or women who are trying to conceive) limit their fat intake. Low-fat foods are not good for fertility as healthy omega-3 fatty acids may assist with preconception due to the effect they have on increased uterine blood flow.[35] In addition, some studies suggest that omega-3 fatty acids found in foods such as wild salmon and egg yolks may also aid with reproductive hormone regulation.[36] Not to mention, monounsaturated fat such as extra-virgin olive oil helps increase insulin sensitivity (meaning you need less

If you or your partner are not gene carriers for the two main genes for celiac disease, that does not rule you out for non-celiac gluten sensitivity (NCGS). It is important to consider eating at least gluten-free, if not some form of a nutritious whole food diet that does not include grains (especially wheat, barley, rye, or contaminated oats) before, during, and after your pregnancy and perhaps for good. Additionally, dairy is typically an issue due to the fact that the gluten and the casein proteins are molecularly very similar and our bodies tend to read these proteins the same. Of course, removing any other foods that you are sensitive to or intolerant to is a great idea, especially while you are pregnant and breastfeeding. A diet that consists of organic fruits and vegetables, meat, fish, and eggs, and of course, high quality fats such as avocadoes, olive oil, and coconut oil is beneficial.

—**Nadine Grzeskowiak, RN, BSN, CEN**

34   J. Chavarro et al., "A prospective study of dietary carbohydrate quantity and quality in relation to risk of ovulatory infertility," NCBI, September 19, 2007, accessed September 13, 2017, https://www.ncbi.nlm.nih.gov/pmc/articles/PMC3066074/.

35   P. Saldeen and T. Saldeen, "Women and omega-3 Fatty acids.," NCBI, October 2004, accessed September 19, 2017, https://www.ncbi.nlm.nih.gov/pubmed/15385858.

36   A. Nadjarzadeh et al., "The effect of omega-3 supplementation on androgen profile and menstrual status in women with polycystic ovary syndrome: A randomized clinical trial," NCBI, August 2013, accessed September 19, 2017, https://www.ncbi.nlm.nih.gov/pmc/articles/PMC3941370/.

insulin to combat blood sugar, which is a good thing!) and reduce inflammation.[37] Once you have conceived, healthy fats are critical for fetal brain, eye, and nervous system development. Keep in mind that not all fats are created equally; it is imperative (for fertility and pregnancy) to severely limit unhealthy fats that are found in items such as fast-foods, fried foods, hot dogs, and hydrogenated vegetable oil.

Synthetic Folic Acid, Folate, and 5-methyltetrahydrofolate

Consuming adequate amounts of folate before you conceive is imperative; folate is a B vitamin that greatly reduces fetal neural tube defects of the brain, spine, and spinal cord. These defects usually occur in the first three weeks after conception so it is best to regularly get your folate for several months before your pregnancy. You may be wondering—isn't folic acid found in a prenatal vitamin the same as folate so can't I just take a pill every day? Technically, yes, some can use synthetic folic acid in the form of a supplement or by eating fortified foods such as cereal, however, it may be far more efficient and beneficial to find naturally occurring folate in whole foods. For your fetus to reap the benefits of folic acid, your body must be able to convert synthetic folic acid into the biologically functional form 5-methyltetrahydrofolate. Not everyone is capable of facilitating this conversion which may lead to levels of folic acid that are not substantial enough for your developing fetus.[38] If you choose to supplement as opposed to getting your folate from naturally occurring foods (found later in this chapter), you may want to discuss with your doctor the possibility of supplementing with 5-methyltetrahydrofolate as opposed to folic acid.

Now let's take a look at the macro- and micro-nutrients you should be consuming along with all of the delicious foods you can find them in. If you are planning to become pregnant in the near future, these are especially vital for all women as they not only have a positive effect on fertility and emotional well-being, but also on the young embryo before you can even detect

---

37   AA Rivellese, DE Natale, and S. Lilli, "Type of dietary fat and insulin resistance.," NCBI, June 2002, accessed September 20, 2017, https://www.ncbi.nlm.nih.gov/pubmed/12079860.

38   R. Obeid, W. Holzgreve, and K. Pietrzik, "Is 5-methyltetrahydrofolate an alternative to folic acid for the prevention of neural tube defects?" NCBI, September 01, 2013, accessed September 11, 2017, https://www.ncbi.nlm.nih.gov/pubmed/23482308.

that you are pregnant. Whether you have no known fertility issues, infertility issues, or specific conditions such as Polycystic Ovary Syndrome, including the following into your daily diet is beneficial during this exciting time!

During the early stages of pregnancy and even prior to conception, optimal nutrition, self-care, exercise, medical and prenatal care, socialization, and adequate sleep can help to ensure that a woman is physically and emotionally prepared to provide the greatest likelihood for a healthy pregnancy, as well as a healthy beginning to the initial phases of motherhood. Maintaining balance in these areas can allow a woman to feel more in control and better prepared for pregnancy, child birth, and motherhood. As a woman transitions into motherhood, she will experience great physical, emotional, and psychological changes. During pregnancy, as well as in life in general, stress is often unavoidable. In those times, an expectant mother may find that taking proper care of her physical and emotional well-being and appropriately coping with stress can help to make pregnancy more enjoyable. From a mental health perspective, it is also important to note that acceptance of stress can allow a woman to feel more in control of her health and of her pregnancy. While taking measures to eliminate stress is important, awareness and acceptance that stress is inevitable and unavoidable may be an essential first step in coping. This can be referred to as mindfulness. Being mindful and allowing one to be present and self-aware can help to make stressors more bearable, particularly during pregnancy. Mindful practices can be simple: being present in the moment, paying attention to breathing and body cues, accepting what a mother is experiencing and feeling, rather than fighting or pushing the feelings away, and being intentional about being present in that moment with those emotions. Utilizing these practices may help to reduce stress and improve mood and overall functioning[39] in day to day life as you begin the journey with your tiny, yet great addition to your life and family.

—Kara Cruz, MA, Registered Associate Marriage and Family Therapist

39 Harvard Health Publishing, "What meditation can do for your mind, mood, and health," Harvard Health, accessed September 12, 2017, https://www.health.harvard.edu/staying-healthy/what-meditation-can-do-for-your-mind-mood-and-health.

Macronutrients

Macronutrients are foods that are required in large amounts (carbohydrates, fats, protein, and fiber). *The Whole Food Pregnancy Plan's* macronutrient philosophy is research-based and results-driven, aiding in the avoidance of many diet-related pregnancy ailments. Incorporating these types of macros into every meal and snack will put you on the path to a nutritionally fit pregnancy.

Low-Glycemic, Gluten-Free Carbohydrates

Function: Low-glycemic carbohydrates provide adequate amounts of energy while keeping blood sugar levels even. Getting in the habit of consuming these types of carbohydrates before conception is key to avoiding sugar-related issues such as gestational diabetes. Also, low-glycemic carbohydrates aid in conception as they do not trigger an insulin response that may inhibit ovulation. Moreover, they are unprocessed and provide more nutrients per calorie than their high-glycemic counterparts.

Omega-3 Fatty Acids

Function: These fats assist in balanced sex hormone production so adequate intake of omega-3 fatty acids (specifically EPA and DHA) could increase your chances of conceiving. Once you have conceived, good fat is imperative for fetal brain, eye, and nervous system development.

Quality Proteins

Function: Protein is one of the essential building blocks for your baby-to-be and choosing organic, grass-fed and wild varieties of chicken, meat, and seafood is critical in order to limit environmental toxins and added hormones that can be found in non-organic versions. If you are vegan or vegetarian, be sure to consume enough protein through plant-based sources such as quinoa, lentils, broccoli, spinach, and nuts.

Fiber

Function: According to an American Journal of Hypertension report, women who increase fiber intake early on in pregnancy are less likely to develop pregnancy-related high blood pressure and preeclampsia.[40] The added fiber will also help to keep you regular!

---

40 C. Qiu et al., "Dietary fiber intake in early pregnancy and risk of subsequent preeclampsia.," NCBI, August 2008, accessed September 19, 2017, https://www.ncbi.nlm.nih.gov/pubmed/18636070.

Micronutrients

If you are trying to conceive, you should be eating a very broad range of all micronutrients (vitamins and minerals). The following list contains ones that have extremely high importance during preconception due to documented deficiencies that tend to be common in pregnant women. Some are also noted for their ability to increase fertility chances while greatly reducing the incidence of certain birth defects in very early stages of pregnancy.

Vitamin B6

All B vitamins are critical during preconception but vitamin B6 stands out as it is known to increase progesterone—a hormone needed to sustain your pregnancy after conception.

Superior Sources: *spinach, cauliflower, sweet potato, garlic, chicken, turkey, wild salmon*

Vitamin C

Your body will be working overtime in the early stages of conception so building a strong immune system (with support from vitamin C) before conception and maintaining it throughout pregnancy is vital. Be sure to keep up with your vitamin C consumption as your immune system may naturally weaken once you are pregnant. Also, pairing foods that contain vitamin with iron sources will maximize iron absorption!

Superior Sources: *bell peppers, broccoli, Brussels sprouts, strawberries, citrus fruits*

Calcium

Like most nutrients, the fetus draws calcium from you, so building your calcium stores before pregnancy is essential. Insufficient calcium intake can result in the breakdown of the maternal bones in order to transfer needed calcium to the fetus.

Superior Sources: *kale, collard greens, oranges, sardines, canned salmon, almonds*

Choline

Not as popular as folate, choline actually provides the same benefits (and sometimes is able to even take the place of folate) with regard to the prevention of neural tube defects. Research has shown that proper choline intake dramatically reduces the occurrence of brain, spine, and spinal cord defects.

Superior Sources: *eggs, shrimp, scallops, liver, wild salmon, cod, chicken, turkey, kale*

Vitamin D

Be sure to optimize your vitamin D levels if you are struggling with infertility (getting your levels checked is easy to do at your doctor's office). It helps increase levels of estrogen and progesterone in women, which assists with menstrual cycle regulation. For men, vitamin D supports sperm count, quality semen, and testosterone levels.[41] Sufficient vitamin D levels have also been associated with favorable conception outcomes in women who undergo in-vitro fertilization (IVF), as well as in women who suffer from polycystic ovarian syndrome (PCOS).[42] Vitamin D deficiency is common in pregnant women and has been linked to premature birth, as well as the occurrence of ailments such as asthma, diabetes, and even cardiovascular disease in their babies, so it is imperative to keep your levels optimal throughout your pregnancy.

Superior Sources: wild salmon, sardines, eggs, sunlight (more vitamin D options and supplementation choices in Chapter 4!)

Iodine

Trace mineral iodine is essential for preconception as it helps to maintain adequate levels of thyroid hormone. Low levels of thyroid hormone can lead to the cessation of ovulation which can cause infertility. Proper iodine intake also supports immune system function, metabolism, and weight management.

Superior Sources: shrimp, cod, navy beans, potatoes (skin on), strawberries, Greek yogurt, cheddar cheese

Iron

According to some studies, lack of iron is associated with irregular and/or limited ovulation as well the overall health of the egg which can create a rate of infertility that is considerably higher than women who consume adequate amounts of iron.[43] Building your iron stores before conception is also important as your baby will use your iron which could lead to a deficiency.

Superior Sources: spinach, beans, lentils, quinoa, wild salmon, clams, oysters, beef, liver

41 E. Lerchbaum and B. Obermayer-Pietsch, "Vitamin D and fertility: a systematic review.," NCBI, May 2012, accessed September 24, 2017, https://www.ncbi.nlm.nih.gov/pubmed/22275473.

42 E. Lerchbaum and T. Rabe, "Vitamin D and female fertility.," NCBI, June 2014, accessed September 24, 2017, https://www.ncbi.nlm.nih.gov/pubmed/24717915.

43 JE Chavarro et al., "Iron intake and risk of ovulatory infertility.," NCBI, November 2006, accessed September 19, 2017, https://www.ncbi.nlm.nih.gov/pubmed/17077236.

Folate

Studies now suggest that adequate folate intake may improve progesterone levels which may help to regulate ovulation, making it easier to conceive.[44] Possibly the most well-known pre-conception nutrient, significant research has also proven that adequate intake of folate greatly reduces neural tube defects—these occur within three to four weeks of conception (before many may even realize they are pregnant) so folate consumption is critical during the months before you conceive.

Superior Sources: *lentils, beans, asparagus, spinach, cauliflower, Brussels sprouts*

Zinc

Zinc plays a key role in conception as it helps to keep your hormones balanced throughout your menstrual cycle which is key for ovulation. Zinc also aids in the production of sperm and mature eggs that are prime for fertilization.

Superior Sources: *sesame and pumpkin seeds, lentils, quinoa, oysters, shrimp, beef, lamb*

Now that you are aware of some of the most essential nutrients, see the following chart for even more preconception and fertility super-foods that contain the above listed nutrients and much more! These foods will have a positive impact on the embryo before you even know you have conceived, and they will be used throughout your entire pregnancy so it's helpful to start shopping for and cooking with them as soon as possible. Learning to incorporate these foods into your meals and snacks will put you on the path to conception and a nutritionally-fit pregnancy.

In Chapter 8, you can find specific food servings recommendations. If you are unfamiliar with some of these foods, please refer to Chapters 17, 18, 19, 20, and 21 for a variety of simple, delicious recipes and meal plans. They are nutritionally sound for the rest of your family as well!

---

44 A. Gaskins et al., "The Impact of Dietary Folate Intake on Reproductive Function in Premenopausal Women: A Prospective Cohort Study," NCBI, September 26, 2012, accessed September 20, 2017, https://www.ncbi.nlm.nih.gov/pmc/articles/PMC3458830/.

FOOD	MACRONUTRIENTS	MICRONUTRIENTS
Low-Glycemic Vegetables (broccoli, asparagus, Brussels sprouts, onion, cauliflower, spinach, kale, artichoke, collard greens, arugula, butter lettuce, romaine, Swiss chard, cabbage, radish)	Carbohydrate	Vitamins A, C, E, and K; chromium, folate, fiber, pantothenic acid, vitamins B1, B2, and B6; manganese, selenium, pantothenic acid, niacin, potassium, phosphorus, choline, copper, omega-3 fatty acids, calcium, and iron.
Starchy Vegetables (sweet potato, squash, pumpkin, parsnip, zucchini)	Carbohydrate	Vitamins A, C, and K; vitamins B1, B2, B3, and B6; beta carotene, copper, folate, iodine, iron, fiber, and phosphorus.
Low-Sugar Fruits (blueberries, blackberries, raspberries, strawberries, apple, apricot, tomato, bell pepper)	Carbohydrate	Vitamins A, C, E, and K, fiber, biotin, molybdenum, copper, potassium, riboflavin, thiamin, manganese, fiber, iodine, vitamins B2 and B6, folate, niacin, phosphorus, carotenoids.
Other Low-Sugar Fruits (avocado, olives)	Fat	Vitamins C, E, and K, fiber, copper, potassium, vitamin B6, folate, omega-3 fatty acids.
Legumes (lentils, peas, black beans, white beans, pinto beans, garbanzo beans, kidney beans)	Carbohydrate & Protein	Vitamins A, C, and K, protein, thiamin, riboflavin, niacin, Vitamins B1 and B6, calcium, iodine, iron, magnesium, phosphorus, potassium, copper, manganese, folate, zinc, and fiber.
Nuts and Seeds (almonds, cashews, pistachios, pecans, macadamia, walnuts, hazelnuts, sesame seeds, pumpkin seeds, chia seeds, quinoa*)	Fat, Protein, & *Carbohydrate	Vitamin E, vitamins B2 and B6, magnesium, zinc, fiber, biotin, copper, phosphorus, calcium, omega-3 fatty acids.
Poultry (organic chicken, duck, turkey)	Protein	Vitamins B2, B3, B6, and B12; niacin, phosphorus, choline, iron, selenium, zinc, phosphorus, choline, and pantothenic acid.
Other Poultry (eggs)	Protein & Fat	Vitamins A, D, E, K; choline, vitamin B12, thiamin, riboflavin, folate, zinc, copper, and selenium.
Fish (wild salmon, halibut, sole, rockfish, mahi mahi, opah, sardines)	Protein and Fat	Vitamin D, vitamins B5, B6, and B12, iodine, magnesium, potassium, niacin, phosphorus, and selenium; omega-3 fatty acids.
Shellfish (oysters, clams, shrimp, mussels, crab, lobster)	Protein and Fat	Vitamin B12, iron, zinc, copper, iodine, omega-3 fatty acids.
Meat (organic grass-fed beef, organic grass-fed lamb, venison, bison)	Protein and Fat	Vitamins B3, B6, and B12; omega-3 fatty acids, selenium, iron, zinc, phosphorus, choline, and pantothenic acid.

Chapter 7
Getting Back to Your Pre-pregnancy Weight Starts with the First Trimester

If you are reading this chapter because you are in your first trimester, congratulations! If you are in the pre-conception phase but just reading ahead, you'll be there soon! One of the most interesting and important facts about the first trimester is that there are no extra calorie needs unless you are underweight at the time of conception. During your first trimester, if you are carrying a singleton, you will require an average of 1800 calories, given the fact that you are in normal weight range. In the future, you will need an average of 350 additional calories (beyond the baseline of 1800) in the second trimester, and an average of an additional 450 calories (beyond the baseline of 1800) in the third trimester.

If you are carrying twins, guidelines say you should consume 300 extra calories per day in the first trimester, 680 extra per day in the second trimester, and 900 extra per day in the third. If you are expecting triplets, you will need an average of 450 extra calories in the first trimester, 1,020 extra in the second trimester, and 1,350 extra in the third trimester. No two women are the same so if you are unsure of how many calories is appropriate for your baseline or added calories, there are free pregnancy calculators that are easily accessible online, or consult with your health care provider.

General caloric recommendations are an average based on "normal weight" women. For more specific details regarding appropriate caloric intake based on body types, the following chart considers your Body Mass Index (BMI) at the beginning of pregnancy. The Body Mass Index is a calculation of weight to height ratio and can indicate if one is underweight, normal weight, overweight, or obese. To calculate your own BMI, please use the following formula (or you can easily access a free BMI calculator online). Please keep in

Weight Gain and Calorie Needs Based on Body Mass Index and Trimester (Singleton)

BMI at Conception	Pregnancy Weight Gain	Daily Caloric Increase
Less than 18.5 (underweight)	28–40 pounds	1st Trimester: 50–200 extra calories per day 2nd Trimester: 300–400 extra calories per day 3rd Trimester: 400–500 extra calories per day
18.5–24.9 (normal weight)	25–35 pounds	1st Trimester: 0 extra calories per day 2nd Trimester: 200–300 extra calories per day 3rd Trimester: 350–450 extra calories per day
25–29.9 (overweight)	15–25 pounds	1st Trimester: 0 extra calories per day 2nd Trimester: 150–200 extra calories per day 3rd Trimester: 250–350 extra calories per day
30 or greater (obese)	11–20 pounds	1st Trimester: 0 extra calories per day 2nd Trimester: 100–200 extra calories per day 3rd Trimester: 200–300 extra calories per day

*BMI = weight in pounds / [height in inches x height in inches] x 703

mind, these guidelines are for women who are carrying a single baby. If you are carrying multiples, you will need even more calories, based on how many babies you are carrying, so please consult your doctor if you are unsure what is right for you.

Interestingly enough, getting back to your pre-pregnancy weight (after your baby is here!) really does depend heavily on the first trimester. The habits formed during the beginning of your pregnancy could very well dictate the habits that continue throughout the rest of your pregnancy. My own experience with pregnancy nutrition is best described as learning how to eat all over again! My body didn't quite feel the same as "normal" (as it shouldn't) so my relationship with food was altered in terms of what I wanted to eat and how much. To put it mildly, cravings are real! The good news is that the correct foods will help to combat them. It may be a struggle at times but try your best to remain within five pounds of your pre-pregnancy weight before you enter the second trimester. If you accomplish this, your odds of gaining appropriate pregnancy weight will greatly increase and you'll be quickly on your way to returning to your pre-pregnancy weight once your baby is here. More importantly, your health and that of your baby will be less likely to be compromised.

To find calorie requirements that are specific to your age, height, weight, activity level, and trimester of pregnancy, you can access free calculators online. You will see there is a wide range when it comes to calorie and macronutrient recommendations; a woman who is 4'11" tall and who weighed 100 pounds before conception will have different needs than a woman who is 5'11" who weighed 165 pounds before conception, so these are general guidelines. Being mindful of calorie amounts is important, however, it is more important to be concerned with the quality of the calories you are consuming during your whole pregnancy. Below is a list of essential vitamins and nutrients (as well as examples of food sources you can find them in) that are vital while you are expecting. These foods are incorporated in your grocery list found in Chapter 3 as well in a variety of recipes found in Chapters 18, 19, 20, and 21.

Nutrient	Function	Food Source
Vitamin A & Beta Carotene (770 mcg)	Promotes bone and teeth growth	Eggs, carrots, spinach, yellow vegetables, green vegetables, broccoli, potatoes, pumpkin, yellow fruits, cantaloupe, liver
Vitamin D (600 IU–2000 IU)*	Supports strong bones and teeth; helps the body use phosphorus and calcium	Fatty fish, eggs, sunshine
Vitamin E (15 mg)	Aids in the formation and use of muscles and red blood cells	Almonds, sunflower seeds, pumpkin seeds, kale, spinach, coconut oil, olive oil, avocado, broccoli, papaya
Vitamin C (85 mg)	Helps body absorb iron and prevents tissue damage; immune system booster	Bell peppers, citrus fruits, dark leafy greens, strawberries, broccoli, tomatoes
Thiamin/B1 (1.4 mg)	Controls nervous system and promotes energy levels	eggs, berries, nuts, pork, sunflower seeds, black beans, lentils, navy beans, green peas, asparagus, spinach, eggplant, romaine lettuce, cremini mushrooms
Riboflavin/B2 (1.4 mg)	Promotes healthy skin, eyesight and energy; helps body to use other B vitamins	Lamb, wild salmon, Greek yogurt, eggs, spinach, liver, almonds, mushrooms, asparagus, turkey

Niacin/B3 (18 mg)	Helps with digestion and nerves; supports healthy skin	Turkey, chicken, mushrooms, green peas, grass-fed beef, wild salmon, chicken, lamb, shrimp
Pyridoxine/B6 (1.9 mg)	Provides morning sickness relief and promotes formation of red blood cells	Chicken, wild salmon, halibut, liver, pork, eggs, carrots, cabbage, cantaloupe, peas, spinach, sunflower seeds, bananas, beans, broccoli, walnuts
Folic Acid/Folate (600–800 mcg)	Helps to prevent neural tube defects and promotes placenta health	Lentils, beans, Brussels sprouts, cauliflower, asparagus, peas, strawberries
Calcium (1,000–1,300 mg)	Develops strong teeth and bones; aids in blood clot prevention and the function of nerves and muscles	Cooked kale, Greek yogurt, kefir, sardines with bones, broccoli, watercress, bok choy, okra, almonds, canned salmon, butternut squash, beans
Choline (450 mg)	Helps to develop nervous system, brain and prevent neural tube defects	Egg yolks, avocado, beef, liver, salmon, cauliflower, Brussels sprouts
Iodine (220 mcg)	Develops nervous system and brain; also regulates metabolism and thyroid gland	Shrimp, cod, strawberries, Greek yogurt, cheddar cheese, navy beans, and potato (skin on)
Iron (27 mg)	Prevents anemia and aids in hemoglobin production; helps to avoid premature delivery and low birth weight	Clams, mussels, beef, sardines, chicken, turkey, halibut, wild salmon, spinach, beans, sesame seeds, pumpkin seeds, peas, broccoli, almonds, walnuts
Fiber (25 g–30 g)	Assists with digest and helps to prevent constipation and high blood pressure	Berries, artichoke hearts, avocado, chia seeds, flaxseed, almonds, beans, lentils, broccoli, Brussels sprouts, figs, quinoa
Protein (75 g–100 g)	Repairs cells and assists in amino acid production; vital for fetal growth and development	Eggs, fish, beef, poultry, shellfish, Greek yogurt, broccoli, lentils, peas, beans, nuts, seeds, quinoa, kale, artichoke, spinach
Omega-3 Fatty Acids, DHA & EPA (1,000 mg)	Greatly contributes to fetal brain, eye, and nervous system development	Fatty fish, oysters, crab, shrimp, seaweed, fish oil, krill oil
Zinc (11–12 mg)	Promotes enzyme and insulin production	Oysters, beef, lamb, sesame seeds, pumpkin seeds, lentils, turkey, quinoa, shrimp

*Some studies suggest that higher intake of vitamin D (as much as 6,400/day IU) is beneficial and safe during pregnancy.[45] Please consult with your doctor regarding the best vitamin D supplementation for you.

---

45   Samar Al Emadi and Mohammed Hammoudeh, "Vitamin D study in pregnant women and their babies," NCBI, November 01, 2013, accessed August 30, 2017, https://www.ncbi.nlm.nih.gov/pmc/articles/PMC3991049/.

Folate Emphasis

You are probably already aware of the importance of folate and even though I already touched on it in previous chapters, I'd like to mention it again. Just a reminder that folate (or synthetic folic acid) is most critical during the first three to four weeks following conception. Neural tube defects of the brain and spine occur during this timeframe so if you just found out you are pregnant or suspect that you may be pregnant, be sure you load up on your folate-rich foods if you are not taking synthetic folic acid. Below is an extensive list of folate-rich foods so you can achieve your minimum of 600 micrograms per day! If you consume more than that, not to worry—our bodies can regulate naturally occurring folate. If you are obtaining your requirement through synthetic folic acid, please do not consume more than 1,000 micrograms per day as that is the established tolerable upper intake level.

Source	Serving Size	Folate Per Serving (mcg)
Lentils	1 Cup	358
Pinto Beans	1 Cup	294
Garbanzo Beans	1 Cup	282
Asparagus (cooked)	1 Cup	262
Black Beans	1 Cup	256
Navy Beans	1 Cup	254
Kidney Beans	1 Cup	230
Okra (cooked)	1 Cup	206
Spinach (cooked)	1 Cup	200
Collard Greens (cooked)	1 Cup	177
Turnip Greens	1 Cup	170
Brussels sprouts (cooked)	1 Cup	160
Spinach (raw)	1 Cup	110
Mustard Greens	1 Cup	103
Green Peas	1 Cup	101
Broccoli (cooked)	1 Cup	100
Sunflower Seeds	¼ Cup	82
Strawberries	8 Medium	80
Beets	½ Cup	74
Cauliflower (cooked)	1 Cup	70
Romaine Lettuce	1 Cup	65
Papaya	½ of a Papaya	58
Avocado	½ Cup	55
Flax Seeds	2 tbsp	54
Green Beans	1 Cup	42
Orange	1 Medium	40

Morning Sickness

Unfortunately, data shows that morning sickness affects over half of all pregnant women—the good news is that morning sickness can possibly be combated with nutrition! Studies have shown that ginger and vitamin B6 aid in the treatment of pregnancy-induced nausea and vomiting (otherwise known as morning sickness).[46] During my own pregnancy, when I started to feel an onset of nausea, I would consume a meal that contained both ginger and B6 and, coincidentally, my morning sickness subsided. After testing this method out three times, I incorporated Vitamin B6-rich foods and ginger into my daily nutrition regimen and sure enough, my morning sickness was either extremely mild or non-existent by week eight of my pregnancy.

There are several Vitamin B6-rich foods to choose from whether you eat animal proteins or not. Consuming Vitamin B6

---

46 E. Haji Seid Javadi, F. Salehi, and O. Mashrabi, "Comparing the Effectiveness of Vitamin B6 and Ginger in Treatment of Pregnancy-Induced Nausea and Vomiting," NCBI, October 22, 2013, accessed September 13, 2017, https://www.ncbi.nlm.nih.gov/pmc/articles/PMC3819920/.

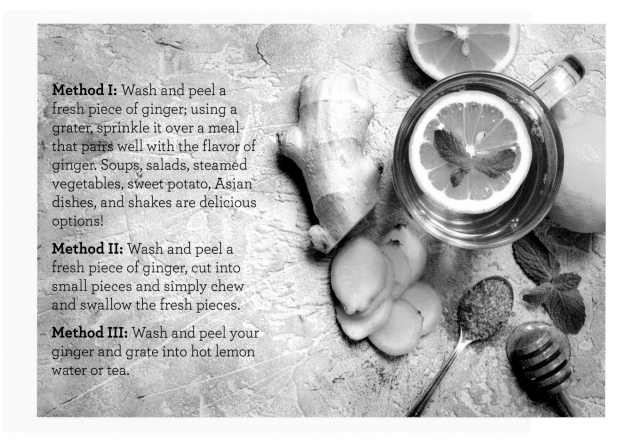

Method I: Wash and peel a fresh piece of ginger; using a grater, sprinkle it over a meal that pairs well with the flavor of ginger. Soups, salads, steamed vegetables, sweet potato, Asian dishes, and shakes are delicious options!

Method II: Wash and peel a fresh piece of ginger, cut into small pieces and simply chew and swallow the fresh pieces.

Method III: Wash and peel your ginger and grate into hot lemon water or tea.

from naturally occurring foods sources has not been determined to lead to toxicity; however, too much Vitamin B6 from supplements can be detrimental so please discuss supplementation with your doctor if that is the route you prefer to take. Some of the best vitamin B6 food sources are sunflower seeds, pistachio nuts, flaxseeds, walnuts, hazelnuts, wild salmon, halibut, turkey, chicken, pork chops, dried prunes, dried apricots, raisins, lean beef, banana, avocado, and cooked spinach.

Boasting Vitamin C, copper, potassium, magnesium, and manganese, ginger has been valued for its medicinal properties in Asia for thousands of years. I prefer fresh ginger root due to its flavor and superior nutrient composition, but powdered ginger is fairly comparable so if that is more convenient then feel free to use that alternative. Ginger has chemicals, phenols, and compounds that perform a variety of functions such as stomach acid neutralization which leads to morning sickness alleviation. According to the American Pregnancy Association, the use of ginger root is "likely safe" during pregnancy. It should not be consumed in large amounts though, so the use of ginger extract is not advised as it is concentrated, resulting in possible side effects. Side

effects from responsible ginger intake are unlikely when limiting ginger intake to 1,000 milligrams per day while you are expecting.

Other tactics I used to fight morning sickness were eating immediately after waking up (an empty stomach can heighten nausea) as well as always having lemons on hand. The smell and taste of freshly cut lemons work well for many people. Even though morning sickness is unpleasant, it is a sign that your pregnancy is progressing and hopefully, it will subside by your second trimester. Hang in there!

Now that we have gone over primary needs of the first trimester, let's put this information to use and incorporate these details into a sample meal plan. Keep in mind that Chapters 17, 18, 19, 20, and 21 provide extensive meal planning ideas and detailed recipes, however, I would like to exhibit an example of a one-day meal plan here that is specific to your folate needs during this time. Consuming a folate-rich diet (at least 600 micrograms per day) at the very beginning of your pregnancy (and ideally, before you conceive) is critical to prevent neural tubal defects. You'll see how simple it is to incorporate foods from this chapter's folate list into your snacks and meals.

Folate quantities for the top sources in each meal are provided; minimal amounts from other foods are not listed.

Breakfast

Gluten-free oatmeal topped with 2 tablespoons of ground flaxseeds (*54 mcg folate*) and eight sliced strawberries (*80 mcg folate*). *Breakfast Folate Total:* 134 micrograms

Lunch

1 cup of chopped Romaine leaves (*65 mcg folate*) topped with sliced chicken breast (omit chicken if you are vegetarian or vegan), ¼ cup garbanzo beans (*71 mcg folate*), ¼ cup green beans (*11 mcg folate*), ½ of a tomato (*10 mcg folate*), and diced onion. Top with extra-virgin olive oil and balsamic vinegar. *Lunch Folate Total:* 157 micrograms

Snack

½ cup mashed avocado (*55 mcg folate*) with your favorite vegetables. *Snack Folate Total:* 55 micrograms

Snack

23 raw almonds (*14 mcg folate*). *Snack Folate Total:* 14 micrograms

Dinner

Using extra-virgin olive oil and your favorite seasonings, grill or pan-cook a six-ounce piece of wild salmon (substitute Tempeh if vegetarian or vegan). Serve with ½ cup cooked lentils (*179 mcg folate*) and ½ cup of cooked Brussels sprouts (*80 mcg folate*). *Dinner Folate Total:* 259 micrograms *Meal Plan Folate Total:* 619 micrograms

See how easy it is to acquire 619 micrograms of folate? Not only does the meal plan exceed the 600 microgram requirement for folate, it offers a variety of other essential micronutrients, low-glycemic carbohydrates, quality proteins, and essential fatty acids—all of which came from whole, unprocessed foods! See you in your second trimester!

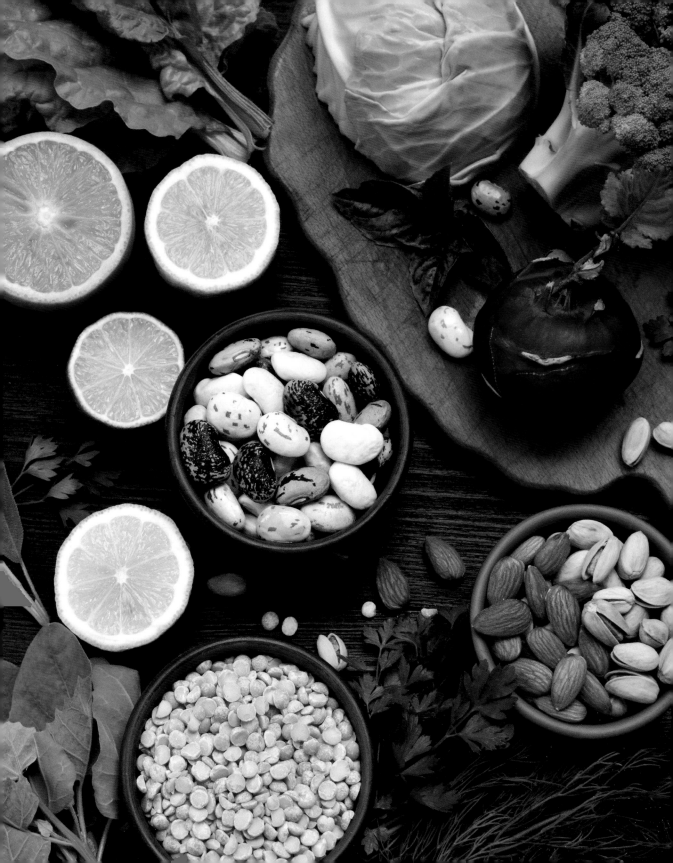

Chapter 8
Food Groups and Servings for All Trimesters

Though there are some particular superstar nutrients that have significant trimester-specific importance (i.e., folate in the first trimester), the food groups and servings exhibited in this chapter can be used throughout your whole pregnancy. One of the only substantial differences to take consideration for each trimester is caloric intake (refer to page 136 for more detailed info about caloric needs per trimester!). Keep in mind, these calorie guidelines are very general averages, as someone who is 4'11" and weighed 95 pounds before pregnancy will have different caloric needs than someone who is 5'11" and weighed 170 pounds before pregnancy.

They types of calories you consume while expecting are just as (if not more) important than the amounts of calories you consume. Due to their macro- and micro-nutrient contents, the following food groups are essential for a healthy pregnancy so I highly recommend making these guidelines an everyday goal to fulfill. It is important to note that you are *not* restricted to the foods listed on the next few pages; these food groups should take priority in your daily regimen; however, you will be able to incorporate other foods as well. (For a complete list of acceptable *Whole Food Pregnancy* foods, please refer to Chapter 3.)

① Low-Glycemic Vegetables (5-8 servings)

Nutrient-dense vegetables are a good source of low-glycemic carbohydrates that will give you energy but help to maintain even blood sugar levels. Several vitamins, such as vitamins A and C, and minerals such as iron and magnesium are also found in these vegetables—plus many are high in calcium and fiber! If you do not see your favorite low-glycemic vegetable below, feel free to include it in your daily food regimen. The average amount of calories, carbohydrates, protein, fat, and fiber for the vegetables I provided are twelve calories, two grams of carbohydrates, one gram of protein, zero grams of fat, and two grams of fiber, in case you would like to compare your vegetable of choice to the ones in the recommended list.

Whether you eat five, six, seven, or eight servings per day will be based on your personal caloric needs. Since everyone is different, you can tailor your green vegetable needs based on your overall caloric intake requirements.

Green Vegetable	Serving Size	Calories	Carbohydrates	Protein	Fat	Fiber
Spinach (cooked)	½ Cup	23	4 grams	3 grams	0 grams	2.5 grams
Broccoli	½ Cup	16	3 grams	1.5 grams	0 grams	1 gram
Kale	½ Cup	17	3 grams	1.5 gram	0 grams	1 gram
Collard Greens	½ Cup	6	1 gram	0.5 grams	0 grams	0.5 grams
Cabbage	½ Cup	9	2 grams	0.5 grams	0 grams	1 gram
Brussels sprouts	½ Cup	19	4 grams	1.5 grams	0 grams	1.5 grams
Bok Choy	½ Cup	5	1 gram	0.5 grams	0 grams	0 grams
Romaine lettuce	½ Cup	8	0.5 grams	0.5 grams	0 grams	0 grams
Arugula	½ Cup	3	0 grams	0 grams	0 grams	0 grams
Cauliflower	½ Cup	13	2.5 grams	1 gram	0 grams	1 gram

② Low-Sugar Fruits (3–4 servings)

Low-sugar fruits are another source of carbohydrates and energy. In addition, they provide even more micronutrients to add to the variety of benefits the low-glycemic vegetables boast. Try to incorporate tomato or red bell pepper in your 3–4 servings of low-sugar fruits as they contain lycopene—lycopene is a powerful antioxidant that is beneficial to pregnant women! If you do not see your favorite low-sugar fruit below, feel free to include it in your daily food regimen—try to stick to fruits that have eight grams of sugar or less per serving. The average amount of calories, carbohydrates, protein, fat, and fiber for the fruits I provided are forty-one calories, seven grams of carbohydrates, one gram of protein, one gram of fat, and two grams of fiber, in case you would like to compare your low-sugar fruit choice to the ones in the recommended list.

Whether you eat three or four servings per day will be based on your personal caloric needs. Since everyone is different, you can tailor your low-sugar fruit needs based on your overall caloric intake requirements.

Low-Sugar Fruit	Serving Size	Calories	Carbohydrates	Protein	Fat	Fiber
Avocado	½ Cup	117	6 grams	1.5 grams	11 grams	5 grams
Tomato	½ Cup	16	3.5 grams	1 gram	0 grams	1 gram
Bell Pepper	½ Cup	15	3.5 grams	0 grams	0 grams	1 gram
Blueberries	½ Cup	43	11 grams	0.5 grams	0 grams	2 grams
Raspberries	½ Cup	33	8 grams	1 gram	0 grams	4 grams
Strawberries	½ Cup	25	6 grams	0.5 grams	0 grams	1.5 grams
Blackberries	½ Cup	31	7 grams	1 gram	0 grams	4 grams
Apricot	½ Cup	39	9 grams	1 gram	0 grams	1.5 grams
Grapefruit	½ Whole Grapefruit	49	13 grams	1 gram	0 grams	2 grams

③ Probiotic Foods (0–2 servings)

Our bodies contain "good" and "bad" bacteria and probiotics are the friendly bacteria which are critical to maintain a healthy gut flora while you are expecting. During pregnancy, the bad bacteria tend to become more prevalent, so consuming good sources of bacteria is beneficial. (For more details about the importance of probiotics, as well as alternatives for supplements, please refer to Chapter 4.) If you do not see your favorite probiotic food below, feel free to include it in your daily food regimen. The average amount of calories, carbohydrates, protein, fat, and fiber for the probiotic foods below are seventy-five calories, 5.5 grams of carbohydrates, 6.5 grams of protein, four grams of fat, and one gram of fiber, in case you would like to compare your own probiotic food choice to the ones in the recommended list.

Whether you eat zero, one, or two servings per day will be based on your personal caloric needs. Since everyone is different, you can tailor your probiotic needs based on your overall caloric intake requirements. When/if choosing Greek yogurt and kefir, be sure to look for the plain options as flavored yogurt can have as much as twenty-two grams of sugar per serving which is comparable to the amount of sugar you will find in ice cream. In addition, the label "live active cultures" assures that your chosen yogurt does contain beneficial probiotics. If you have aversions to the above-listed probiotic food sources, feel free to skip them but you may want to consider a probiotic supplement.

Probiotic Foods	Serving Size	Calories	Carbohydrates	Protein	Fat	Fiber
Plain Whole Fat Greek Yogurt	½ Cup	110	5 grams	13 grams	5 grams	0 grams
Plain 2% Greek Yogurt	½ Cup	90	5 grams	11 grams	2.5 grams	0 grams
Plain Whole Fat Kefir	½ Cup	80	6 grams	4.5 grams	4.5 grams	0 grams
Plain 2% Kefir	½ Cup	55	6 grams	4.5 grams	2 grams	0 grams
Coconut Milk Kefir	½ Cup	25	2 grams	0.5 gram	2.5 grams	0 grams
Tempeh	½ Cup	160	8 grams	15.5 grams	9 grams	7 grams
Natto	½ Cup	186	12.5 grams	15.5 grams	9.5 grams	4.5 grams
Apple Cider Vinegar	1 tbsp.	3	0 grams	0 grams	0 grams	0 grams
Brine-cured Olives	6 large olives	30	2 grams	0 grams	3 grams	0.5 gram
Sauerkraut	½ cup	14	3 grams	0.5 gram	0 grams	2 grams

④ Starchy Produce (0–2 servings/day)

Starchy produce is another source of carbohydrates that contain essential nutrients. The following foods are higher in carbohydrates so we recommend eating fewer servings than low-glycemic vegetables; however, adding some servings of starchy produce (a few days per week) will increase the variety of antioxidants and nutrients in your diet. If you do not see your favorite starchy produce below, feel free to include it in your food regimen. The average amount of calories, carbohydrates, protein, fat, and fiber for the starches I provided are forty-six calories, thirteen grams of carbohydrates, one gram of protein, zero grams of fat, and 1.5 grams of fiber, in case you would like to compare your starchy produce choice to the ones in the recommended list.

Starchy Produce	Serving Size	Calories	Carbohydrates	Protein	Fat	Fiber
Sweet Potato	½ Cup	57	18 grams	1 gram	0 grams	2 grams
Fingerling Potatoes	4 fingerling Potatoes	100	25 grams	4 grams	0 grams	3 grams
Acorn Squash	½ Cup	28	8 grams	0.5 gram	0 grams	1 gram
Butternut Squash	½ Cup	32	8 grams	1 gram	0 grams	1.5 grams
Pumpkin	½ Cup	15	4 grams	0.5 gram	0 grams	0 grams

⑤ Protein (3-5 servings)

Protein is an essential building block for your baby's development, but not all proteins are created equal. It is imperative to consume high quality proteins (organic if possible) that are unprocessed and have minimal preservatives, fillers, and environmental toxins. If you eat animal proteins, be sure to incorporate a balance of both plant and animal proteins when choosing your options (for example, a dinner consisting of three ounces of chicken, ½ cup of cooked lentils, and a side salad will be a proper balance of two servings of protein). If you do not see your favorite protein below, feel free to include it in your daily food regimen. The average amount of calories, carbohydrates, protein, fat, and fiber for the proteins I provided are 107 calories, seven grams of carbohydrates, eleven grams of protein, four grams of fat, and three grams of fiber, in case you would like to compare your protein choice to the ones in the recommended list.

The number of servings you eat per day will be based on your personal caloric needs. Since everyone is different, you can tailor your protein needs based on your overall caloric intake requirements. If you add your own protein to the list, be sure to avoid low-quality choices that have detrimental additives such as nitrates; items such as hot dogs, deli meats, and fast food meats should be eliminated.

Protein	Serving Size	Calories	Carbohydrates	Protein	Fat	Fiber
Eggs	1 Whole Egg (large)	78	0.5 grams	6 grams	5 grams	0 grams
Chicken (boneless/skinless)	3 ounces	90	0 grams	17 grams	1.5 grams	0 grams
Turkey (breast without skin)	3 ounces	120	0 grams	26 grams	1 gram	0 grams
Cod	3 ounces	70	0 grams	15 grams	1 gram	0 grams
Shrimp	3 ounces	90	1 gram	17 grams	1.5 grams	0 grams
Scallops	3 ounces	90	5 grams	17 grams	0.5 gram	0 grams
Wild Salmon	3 ounces	143	0 grams	18 grams	8 grams	0 grams
Lean grass-fed beef	3 Ounces	158	0 grams	26 grams	5 grams	0 grams
Venison	3 Ounces	128	0 grams	25 grams	2 grams	0 grams
Tempeh	½ Cup	160	8 grams	15.5 grams	9 grams	7 grams
Natto	½ Cup	186	12.5 grams	15.5 grams	9.5 grams	4.5 grams
Quinoa	½ Cup (cooked)	111	20 grams	4 grams	4 grams	5 grams
Black Beans	½ Cup (cooked)	113	20 grams	8 grams	0 grams	7 grams
Lentils	½ Cup (cooked)	115	20 grams	9 grams	0 grams	8 grams
Raw Almonds	23 Whole Almonds	163	6 grams	6 grams	14 grams	3.5 grams
Raw Walnuts	14 halves	185	4 grams	4 grams	18 grams	2 grams
Ground Flax Seeds	2 Tbsp. (ground)	74	4 grams	3 grams	6 grams	4 grams
Chia Seeds	2 Tbsp.	138	12 grams	5 grams	9 grams	10 grams
Hemp Seeds	2 Tbsp.	81	5 grams	10.5 grams	5 grams	3 grams
Spinach (cooked)	½ Cup	23	4 grams	3 grams	0 grams	2.5 grams
Broccoli	1 Cup	31	6 grams	3 grams	0 grams	2.5 grams
Kale	1 Cup	33	6 grams	3 grams	0.5 grams	1.5 grams
Artichoke	½ Medium Artichoke	30	6.5 grams	2 grams	0 grams	3.5 grams
Gluten-free Oatmeal	1 Cup (cooked)	158	27 grams	6 grams	3 grams	4 grams

⑥ Healthy Fats (3-4 servings)

This group contains the beneficial fats that are critical for fetal brain development, as well as maternal health. We will focus on monounsaturated fats as well as polyunsaturated fats such as omega-3 fatty acids as consuming these as opposed to trans-fatty acids is known to positively affect cholesterol levels; also, studies suggest healthy fats improve the brain function of the fetus.[47] The average amount of calories, carbohydrates, protein, fat, and fiber for the healthy fats below are 101 calories, three grams of carbohydrates, 5.5 grams of protein, eight grams of fat, and 1.5 grams of fiber.

How much you eat per day will be based on your personal caloric needs. Since everyone is different, you can tailor your healthy fat needs based on your overall caloric intake requirements.

Healthy Fat	Serving Size	Calories	Carbohydrates	Protein	Fat	Fiber
Avocado	½ Cup	117	6 grams	1.5 grams	11 grams	5 grams
Raw Walnuts	14 halves	185	4 grams	4 grams	18 grams	2 grams
Wild Salmon	3 ounces	143	0 grams	18 grams	8 grams	0 grams
Eggs	1 Whole Egg (large)	78	0.5 grams	6 grams	5 grams	0 grams
Chia Seeds	1 Tbsp.	69	6 grams	2.5 grams	4.5 grams	5 grams
Ground Flax Seeds	1 Tbsp.	30	4 grams	1.5 grams	2.5 grams	3 grams
Extra-Virgin Olive Oil	1 Tsp.	40	0 grams	0 grams	5 grams	0 grams
Coconut Oil	1 Tsp.	39	0 grams	0 grams	4.5 grams	0 grams
Avocado Oil	1 Tsp.	40	0 grams	0 grams	4.5 grams	0 grams
Raw Almonds	23 Whole Almonds	163	6 grams	6 grams	14 grams	3.5 grams
Raw Cashews	18 Whole Cashews	157	9 grams	5 grams	12 grams	1 gram
Raw Almond Butter	1 Tbsp.	98	3 grams	3 grams	9 grams	2 grams
Raw Cashew Butter	1 Tbsp.	94	4 grams	3 grams	8 grams	0 grams
Lean grass-fed beef	3 Ounces	158	0 grams	26 grams	5 grams	0 grams

47   J. Rombaldi Bernardi et al., "Fetal and Neonatal Levels of Omega-3: Effects on Neurodevelopment, Nutrition, and Growth," NCBI, October 17, 2017, , accessed September 24, 2017, https://www.ncbi.nlm.nih.gov/pmc/articles/PMC3483668/.

⑦ Cheat Foods (0–1 Serving)

Back in Chapter 2 we talked about the "90/10 rule," which states that if 90 percent of all of your calories come from the above nutritious sources then you will have some wiggle room to cheat a little bit while still remaining in good nutrition standing with your overall food regimen. If you have a craving that must be satisfied (it happens to all of us!), feel free to allocate 10 percent of your calories to cheat foods. For example, if you are consuming 2,000 calories per day, 10 percent of those calories can be used for whatever you like. Two hundred calories (10 percent of your 2,000) is equivalent to one scoop of ice cream, four small cookies, or one small slice of pizza. Although I do not recommend cheating every single day, if you keep your portion down to 200 calories, you are likely to remain nutritionally healthy.

During my own pregnancy, I tended to "save" up my cheat calories for special occasions. If I knew I would be going to dinner at a restaurant that had my favorite dessert, I would go for three or four days without consuming any cheat calories so I could indulge in my favorite 600-calorie chocolate lava cake! How you divide up your cheat calories is up to you!

If you're unsure of how to incorporate these foods into a meal plan, the following chapter is for you. I'll show you a variety of ways to meet the above recommended servings in two different seven-day meal plans in the following chapter. There will be one-week plans for both non-vegans and vegans, and if you want to get even more creative, *The Whole Food Pregnancy Plan* breakfast, lunch, and dinner recipes found in Chapters 18, 19, and 20 include a variety of these foods.

Chapter 9
Sample Meal Plans

Now that I have talked about daily servings of specific food groups, I'll put these guidelines together in a sample meal plan so you can see what a realistic week of food looks like for both non-vegans and vegans. The meals and snacks found in these plans are meant to be simple with a low number of ingredients and fast preparation times. For more variety, feel free to substitute any meal or snack with recipes found in Chapters 17, 18, 19, 20, and 21.

No beverages are listed with your meals—I highly recommend consuming water (at least eighty ounces per day) as your primary beverage since your blood volume is expanding. Other suitable beverages include unsweetened coffee, tea, mineral water, and water infused with fresh fruits. The American Pregnancy Association recommends consuming no more than 200 milligrams of caffeine per day. Soda, sports drinks, fruit juices, and other sweetened beverages should be eliminated or limited.

Your one-week sample meal plan does not include calories or portion sizes—please adjust portions based on your calorie needs. Also, keep in mind that the following plan is a guide of suggestions; if you dislike a selection of food or have an allergy, please do not consume that particular food—just make a reasonable substitution. The first sample meal plan is for those who consume animal proteins and the second sample meal plan is for vegans.

One Week Meal Plan (Non-Vegan)

DAY (1)

Breakfast: Two- or three-egg omelet with your favorite additions (onion, bell pepper, mushroom, spinach, avocado, grated cheese).

Snack: Greek yogurt topped with favorite berries.

Lunch: Canned chunk-light tuna mixed with diced celery, onions, and tomatoes, topped with freshly squeezed lemon.

Snack: Handful of raw almonds or cashews.

Dinner: Grilled boneless/skinless chicken breast, Brussels sprouts, and sweet potato.

DAY (2)

Breakfast: Oatmeal topped with favorite berries.

Snack: One slice of cheese.

Lunch: Lettuce Wrap "Sandwiches"—two large lettuce cups (iceberg works the best to keep everything together) filled with your favorite protein (chicken, turkey, beef, beans, quinoa, etc.), tomatoes, onions, avocado, and mustard.

Snack: Celery sticks dipped in hummus.

Dinner: Grilled wild salmon with broccoli and mashed cauliflower (steam small head of cauliflower until tender and mash with grated Parmesan cheese).

DAY (3)

Breakfast: One protein pancake (mash one ripe banana with two eggs, combine well and pan-cook in a drizzle of extra-virgin olive oil); top with cinnamon.

Snack: Celery dipped in real peanut or almond butter.

Lunch: Spinach salad (or any greens if you don't like spinach) topped with grilled chicken, red onion, tomato, avocado, walnuts, goat cheese, and a drizzle of extra virgin olive oil and balsamic vinegar.

Snack: Hard-boiled egg.

Dinner: Lean steak with two sides of your favorite green vegetables.

DAY ④

Breakfast: Banana-nut shake (blend ½ banana with handful of ice, one tablespoon of chia seeds, and one tablespoon of real peanut or almond butter).

Snack: Carrot sticks dipped in hummus or guacamole.

Lunch: Salmon Salad—can of wild salmon on bed of greens and favorite salad add-ons (tomatoes, onions, bell peppers, etc.) Top with extra-virgin olive oil, balsamic vinegar, and fresh lemon.

Snack: Handful of blueberries.

Dinner: Mexican Platter—grilled chicken with your favorite seasonings, black beans topped with grated cheese, shredded cabbage, sliced avocado, dollop of Greek yogurt, and Pico de Gallo or salsa.

DAY ⑤

Breakfast: Kale Avocado Shake—blend 1 small banana (very ripe), ½ of an avocado, ½ cup of kefir (milk or almond milk works too) a handful of chopped kale, and a handful of ice cubes.

Snack: Handful of raw almonds.

Lunch: High protein soup (some recommendations are split pea, chicken and vegetable, black bean, and lentil) and green salad topped with sliced tomatoes, onion, avocado, extra-virgin olive oil, and balsamic vinegar.

Snack: ½ grapefruit.

Dinner: Grilled turkey burger and side of your favorite green vegetables; add-ons could include mustard, cheese, avocado, tomato, onion.

DAY ⑥

Breakfast: Protein oatmeal—whisk two egg whites with two tablespoons water, bring to a boil, and cook oatmeal over medium heat until cooked through. Top with favorite berries.

Snack: Your favorite vegetables dipped in hummus.

Lunch: Protein packed salad—greens topped with tomatoes, red onion, garbanzo beans, avocado, extra-virgin olive oil, balsamic vinegar, and your favorite protein (some examples are chicken, turkey, lean beef, shrimp, tuna, fish, beans, lentils).

Snack: Celery dipped in peanut butter.

Dinner: Guilt Free Spaghetti—Preheat oven to 400° F; cut the spaghetti squash in half and remove the seeds. Lightly coat the flesh side with extra-virgin olive oil and your favorite seasonings and place the two halves, flesh-side down, on a lined baking sheet. Bake for 45 minutes to one hour and then use a fork to shred the inside of the squash to get your "noodles." Top with hearty spaghetti sauce (a suggestion is tomato sauce with ground chicken or turkey, bell peppers, onions, mushrooms, and garlic topped with grated Parmesan).

DAY ⑦

Breakfast: Two- or three-egg omelet with your favorite additions (some suggestions are onion, bell pepper, mushroom, spinach, avocado, grated cheese). Use extra-virgin olive oil to sauté your omelet additions as well as your eggs.

Snack: Two small apricots.

Lunch: Lettuce wrap sandwiches—fill large romaine, butter, or iceberg lettuce leaves with your favorite sandwich additions and then fold the lettuce leaves, roll, and cut in half just as you would do with a burrito. Some filling suggestions are turkey, chicken, shrimp, beans, lentils, hummus, sliced tomato, onion, avocado, and mustard.

Snack: Handful of raw almonds or cashews.

Dinner: Grilled boneless pork chops paired with applesauce (check ingredient label to make sure the only ingredient is apple) with a side of your favorite green vegetables.

One Week Meal Plan (Vegan)

DAY ①

Breakfast: Blueberry-Chia Quinoa Oatmeal: Combine ¼ cup quinoa with one cup unsweetened almond milk and ½ mashed banana and cook over medium-low heat until the quinoa is cooked through. Fold in a handful of blueberries and a tablespoon of chia seeds during the last two minutes of cooking.

Snack: Handful of raw almonds or cashews.

Lunch: Hummus and Lentil Lettuce Cups: Mix cooked lentils with desired amount of hummus and place in butter lettuce leaves. Top with chopped green onions and tomato.

Snack: Celery sticks dipped in peanut or almond butter.

Dinner: Tempeh Mexican Platter: Crumble and cook your tempeh according to package instructions, using a drizzle of extra-virgin olive oil and your favorite seasonings. Serve tempeh on a plate with black beans, sliced avocado, shredded cabbage and salsa.

DAY ②

Breakfast: Green Smoothie: In a blender, combine ½ banana, ½ avocado, handful of curly kale, almond or coconut milk, ice, and tablespoon of chia or ground flax seeds.

Snack: Sliced cucumbers dipped in coconut yogurt, topped with pecans or pine nuts.

Lunch: Quinoa Salad: Toss ½ cup cooked quinoa with one teaspoon apple cider vinegar, dried cranberries, and crushed walnuts. Place on a bed of chopped romaine lettuce and top with sliced green onions, avocado, and a drizzle of extra-virgin olive oil.

Snack: Your favorite vegetables dipped in hummus.

Dinner: ½ baked sweet potato topped with garbanzo beans and a drizzle of tahini; pair with a side of steamed broccoli topped with freshly squeezed lemon juice.

DAY ③

Breakfast: Tempeh Scramble: Using a drizzle extra-virgin olive oil and your favorite seasonings, sauté sliced onions and bell peppers for five minutes; add sliced mushrooms to the pan and cook for a few more minutes until everything is somewhat tender. Add crumbled tempeh and continue to cook for three minutes. Stir in halved cherry tomatoes and serve.

Snack: ½ grapefruit.

Lunch: Bean Trio Salad: Combine garbanzo, pinto, and black beans in a bowl and toss with extra-virgin olive oil, apple cider vinegar, freshly squeezed lemon, minced garlic, and chopped cilantro.

Snack: Handful of raw nuts.

Dinner: Spaghetti Squash with Hearty Marinara: Preheat oven to 400° F; cut the spaghetti squash in half and remove seeds. Lightly coat the flesh side with extra-virgin olive oil and your favorite seasonings and place the two halves, flesh-side down, on a lined baking sheet. Bake for 45 minutes to one hour and then use a fork to shred the inside of the squash to get your "noodles." Meanwhile, sauté onions, bell peppers, and mushrooms until tender and combine with marinara sauce over medium heat; top "noodles" with sauce and serve.

DAY ④

Breakfast: Yogurt Parfait: Top almond or coconut yogurt with fresh berries, chia seeds, and crushed walnuts.

Snack: Half an avocado topped with sunflower seeds and a drizzle of agave.

Lunch: Split pea soup (low sodium) paired with green salad topped with tomatoes, onions, a drizzle of extra-virgin olive oil, and balsamic vinegar.

Snack: Baked Kale Chips: Remove stems and roughly chop curly kale. Evenly massage extra-virgin olive oil into leaves and toss with powdered garlic and black pepper. Bake at 350° F for 10–13 minutes or until edges are slightly browned.

Dinner: Natto Cauliflower Rice: Steam a small head of cauliflower until moderately tender (around 15 minutes). Meanwhile, mix natto with a dash or two of tamari and combine until you have a gooey texture. Once the cauliflower is done steaming, use a fork to shred it to create a rice texture. Top your hot cauliflower rice with the prepared Natto and sliced green onions.

DAY ⑤

Breakfast: Gluten-free rolled oatmeal topped with ground flaxseed and sliced strawberries.

Snack: Handful of raw nuts.

Lunch: Sliced tomatoes drizzled with extra-virgin olive oil and balsamic vinegar; top with diced avocado, chopped basil, black pepper, and pinch of salt.

Snack: Your favorite vegetables dipped in hummus.

Dinner: Tempeh strips with Tahini Dip: Cut tempeh into strips and pan-cook or grill with your favorite seasonings for 5–7 minutes. Pair with tahini dip and steamed broccoli topped with freshly squeezed lemon. For dip, combine a tablespoon of tahini with a dollop of whole grain mustard, drizzle of real maple syrup, and enough water to create desired consistency.

DAY ⑥

Breakfast: Ginger-Coconut Chia Seed Pudding: Mash ½ banana and mix with ½ cup unsweetened coconut milk. Combine one tablespoon whole chia seeds into the mixture and refrigerate for one hour or until thickened. Top with freshly grated ginger (optional).

Snack: Baked Parsnip Chips: Slice parsnips into chips (⅛-inch thickness) and toss in extra-virgin olive oil and your favorite seasonings. Bake for 30 minutes at 350° F, turning chips over after the first 15 minutes.

Lunch: BLTA Lettuce Wrap: In one or two large lettuce leaves of your choice, place two tablespoons of Baba Ganoush, two slices of tomato, and two slices of avocado in each lettuce cup and enjoy as a wrap. Baba Ganoush is a mixture of eggplant and tahini and can be found already prepared in most major grocery stores.

Snack: Jicama Sticks with Black Bean Dip: In a food processor or blender, combine black beans, with one teaspoon extra-virgin olive oil, garlic, minced onion, cilantro, fresh lime juice, and enough water to created desired consistency. Pair with sticks of jicama (or your favorite dipping vegetables).

Dinner: High-Protein Broccoli Salad: Slice broccoli florets into bite-sized pieces and place in a large bowl with diced red onion, sesame seeds, and minced dried cranberries or currants. To prepare dressing, mix two tablespoons tahini with a drizzle of maple syrup and dollop of whole grain mustard; add water until you have reached desired consistency. Thoroughly toss the broccoli salad with dressing and serve. Substitute avocado oil mayonnaise (a.k.a. paleo mayo) for dressing for shorter preparation time.

DAY ⑦

Breakfast: Pancakes: Whisk three tablespoons ground flaxseed with seven tablespoons water and set aside in the refrigerator for twenty minutes to thicken. Mash ¾ large banana with a fork in a small mixing bowl and combine with the flaxseed/water mixture until you have a batter-like consistency. Using extra-virgin olive oil, cook your pancakes over medium heat until cooked through (2 minutes on each side). Top with cinnamon.

Snack: Handful of raw nuts of choice.

Lunch: Creamy Cucumber Salad: Combine ½ cup plain almond or coconut yogurt with one sliced green onion, fresh dill, black pepper, and minced garlic. Thoroughly combine with ½ cup thinly sliced cucumbers.

Snack: Baked Kale Chips: Remove stems and roughly chop curly kale. Evenly massage extra virgin olive oil into leaves and toss with powdered garlic and black pepper. Bake at 350°F for 10–13 minutes or until edges are slightly browned.

Dinner: Pecan-Peach Spinach Salad: Toss one cup raw spinach leaves with extra-virgin olive oil and balsamic vinegar until evenly coated. Top with ½ cup cooked quinoa, slices of fresh peach, and pecan halves.

For extended meal planning assistance, you can refer to Chapter 17: The Busy Mom's Meal Planning System. The variety of food choices found in the meal planning system provides flexibility with regard to food preferences, aversions, and nutrition lifestyles. In addition, they are intended to be fairly simple and have shorter preparation times. If you prefer more exploratory recipes, simply choose any breakfast, lunch, and dinner recipes from Chapters 18, 19, and 20 and incorporate your favorite snacks in between.

Chapter 10
Gestational Diabetes

Gestational diabetes affects millions of pregnant women and their babies every year. Research shows that these pregnancy-related conditions may be prevented and/or treated through good nutrition and exercise. Since gestational diabetes is on the rise, it is imperative to take precautions as early as possible—ideally before you conceive! If you are reading this chapter because you have been diagnosed with the condition, I have specialized nutrition guidelines for you.

First of all, what is gestational diabetes? Diagnosed during pregnancy, gestational diabetes results in blood sugar levels that are too high. Ideally, when you eat, the digestive system will covert food into glucose (sugar). The sugar is used for fuel by your cells after it enters the bloodstream. Your pancreas secretes insulin so it can assist with the absorption of the glucose. If your pancreas does not release enough insulin, too much sugar will remain in your blood as opposed to relocating to your cells and being used for energy.

During pregnancy, glucose is needed to nourish your baby so logically, your body becomes a bit more resistant to insulin in order to provide nourishment to your baby.[48] Usually, this will not create an issue as your pancreas knows to secrete additional insulin to process extra sugar found in your bloodstream. In some cases, the pancreas is unable to release enough insulin to keep up with the excess sugar in the blood and therefore, blood sugar levels increase as the sugar is not being converted to energy and used by the cells—this is what results in gestational diabetes!

If you are diagnosed with gestational diabetes, please follow your doctor's orders and get immediate treatment as it can be very dangerous to mother and baby if it goes unrecognized. The

---

48 A. Sonagra et al., "Normal Pregnancy—A State of Insulin Resistance," NCBI, November 2014, accessed September 24, 2017, https://www.ncbi.nlm.nih.gov/pmc/articles/PMC4290225/.

good news is gestational diabetes will dissipate once the baby is born and it is likely that your blood sugar will return to normal levels. There are some risk factors associated with the development of gestational diabetes but keep in mind that not everyone exhibits these risk factors. Several factors are associated with those who are more likely to develop gestational diabetes such as being overweight, being of advanced maternal age, having Polycystic Ovarian Syndrome, having had gestational diabetes before, having a close relative who has been diagnosed with diabetes, or even taking certain medications (consult your doctor). It is important to remember that someone who does not fall into any of the risk factor categories can still develop gestational diabetes so it is best to follow a nutrition plan that will help to prevent it in the first place or treat it after diagnosis.

You may be wondering what to eat to prevent gestational diabetes from occurring. All of the nutrition information outlined in previous and following chapters will help to lower your risk of developing the condition. During my own pregnancy, I refrained from eating gluten 90 percent of the time (no one is perfect,

and who doesn't love a piece of pizza now and then?!) even though I do not have any sort of gluten intolerance. People noticed how I was abstaining from eating items such as bread, pasta, cereal, and crackers during my pregnancy, leading them to ask me if I was gluten-intolerant. I explained that since I was a woman of "advanced maternal age" (over thirty-five years old), I was at higher risk than usual for gestational diabetes so I limited or eliminated all items that were high in sugar or high in carbohydrates that would convert into sugar. The majority of these items, coincidentally, contain gluten so because of that association, I would not consume gluten containing items—it had nothing to do with an intolerance. Some asked me if what I was doing was unhealthy since I was "not eating any carbs." That is probably one of the biggest misconceptions about avoiding things like bread and pasta—the assumption is that if you do not eat those foods then you do not eat any carbohydrates. I recommend that all people eat carbohydrates (pregnant or not)—we need them to survive! Not all carbohydrates demonstrate the same qualities and the effects they have on the human body so it is imperative to select the best carbohydrates possible. Below are some questions to ask yourself to help you identify which carbohydrate-containing foods are most beneficial during your pregnancy and beyond.

- Does the ingredient label on the food exhibit a long list?
  If the answer is yes, it is best to avoid this carbohydrate-containing food. A long ingredient list is a strong indicator that the food is manufactured to a point of being far from a natural state, containing several toxic ingredients.
- Does the food have a shelf life?
  If the answer is yes, it is best to avoid this carbohydrate-containing food. Foods that have a shelf life (such as pasta, bread, crackers, chips, cookies, and cereal) tend to contain a variety of preservatives in order to create that long shelf life.
- Is the food highly processed?
  If the answer is yes, it is best to avoid this carbohydrate-containing food. Processed foods (which are also likely to have long shelf lives) also tend to have a long ingredient list—most of which we can't even pronounce; they are not real foods that occur in nature. Not only do these foods have detrimental additives and preservatives, they

boast inferior fortified nutrients which have been added in the factory and do not absorb well.
- Does the food have added sugar?
  If the answer is yes, it is best to avoid this carbohydrate-containing food. Carbohydrates automatically turn into sugar when digested so it is important not to add to that sugar that will naturally convert in your bloodstream. Keep in mind that there are over 60 different names for sugar that have been found on food labels; some of the most common ones are barley malt, dextrose, rice syrup, sucrose, and high-fructose corn syrup.

The carbohydrate-containing foods I recommend do not fall into any of the above-mentioned categories. They are nutrient-dense whole foods that are unprocessed with little to no shelf lives and have no added sugars. On the next page is a snapshot of some of my favorite carbohydrate foods, based on micronutrient composition and the effect they have on blood sugar levels. I also included carbohydrate foods that we recommend limiting or eliminating for your convenience.

You may be wondering why the whole wheat versions of bread, pasta, crackers, and flour are on the list to avoid since

Carbohydrate Foods to Consume		
Quinoa	Artichoke	Apricot
Acorn Squash	Broccoli	Grapefruit
Butternut Squash	Kale	Tomato
Sweet Potato (boiled)	Brussels Sprouts	Avocado
Fingerling Potatoes (boiled)	Strawberries	Lentils
Pumpkin	Blueberries	Beans
Chia Seeds	Raspberries	
Gluten-Free Oatmeal	Blackberries	

Carbohydrate Foods to Limit or Eliminate		
White Bread	Pizza Crust	Sugary Drinks
Whole Wheat Bread	Croissants	Candy
White Pasta	Muffins	Cookies
Whole Wheat Pasta	Pita Bread	Cake
Cereal	White Flour	Donuts
White Crackers	Whole Wheat Flour	Ice Cream
Tortilla	Bagels	
Commercial Granola Bars	Multi-grain/Whole Wheat Crackers	

these counterparts are touted as items that should be consumed to avoid and/or treat gestational diabetes. The truth of the matter is there is little difference between two pieces of white bread and two pieces of whole wheat bread with regard to their ingredients and nutritional make-up. Let's compare one leading brand of white bread to one leading brand of wheat bread so we can see the similarities (see next page).

	White Bread	Wheat Bread
Serving Size	2 Pieces (52 grams)	2 Pieces (52 grams)
Calories	150	120
Fat	2 grams	1.5 grams
Carbohydrates	28 grams	24 grams
Protein	4 grams	6 grams
Sodium	180 milligrams	220 milligrams
Fiber	1.5 grams	3 grams
Most Abundant Ingredients per Nutrition Label	Enriched bleached flour (wheat flour, malted barley flour), water, high-fructose corn syrup	Whole wheat flour, water, high-fructose corn syrup, wheat, gluten, yeast

As you can see, there is very little difference between the white and wheat bread. It's thought that since wheat bread has double the amount of fiber, it will not affect blood sugar levels negatively, but that is false. That measly extra 1.5 grams of fiber will not make a substantial difference with regard to keeping your blood sugar levels even, especially when combatting twenty-four grams of high-glycemic carbohydrates and high-fructose corn syrup. Fiber does slow down the digestion of carbohydrates which helps to maintain even blood sugar levels. When preventing or managing gestational diabetes, we need foods that have a much higher fiber to carbohydrate ratio than items such as whole wheat bread. Below we compare the amounts of different foods we must eat in order to obtain thirty grams of fiber.

FOOD	Amount of calories you must eat to get 30 grams of fiber	Amount of carbohydrates you must eat to get 30 grams of fiber	Amount of sodium you must eat to get 30 grams of fiber
Whole Wheat Bread	1,350 calories	270 grams	2025 milligrams
Multi-grain Cereal	1,275 calories	275 grams	2,300 milligrams
Whole Wheat Pasta	1,260 calories	246 grams	20 milligrams
Artichoke Hearts	200 calories	45 grams	200 milligrams
Raspberries	240 calories	56 grams	4 milligrams
Chia Seeds	385 calories	33 grams	13 milligrams

The above examples of whole foods are far superior when it comes to their fiber to carbohydrate ratio and will substantially help to prevent or manage gestational diabetes. In addition, they contain a variety of micronutrients that are naturally occurring within the food, and therefore absorb more efficiently. You also will not have to worry about consuming undesirable, hidden ingredients such as high-fructose corn syrup.

More examples of foods that have a high ratio of fiber to carbohydrates that are whole, unprocessed foods are:

Peas, lentils, black beans, Lima beans, broccoli, Brussels sprouts, blackberries, avocado, pears, figs, okra, acorn squash, garbanzo beans, hummus, almonds, flax seeds, quinoa, pomegranate seeds, kiwi, pumpkin seeds, prunes

If you have been diagnosed with gestational diabetes and your doctor said you can manage with proper nutrition, I have put together the following recommendations for you. There are some cases of gestational diabetes that do require medication so please follow your doctor's orders. If you are currently trying to combat gestational diabetes or you have a history of gestational diabetes and you are taking preventative measures, the below guidelines may assist you:

(1) **Severely limit sugar:** The reality of fighting or avoiding gestational diabetes comes down to severely limiting sugar. Consuming sugar is directly related with raising our blood sugar which can result in or exacerbate gestational diabetes. Whether the sugar comes from a candy bar, ice cream, cookies, or even natural sources like honey or fruit, all types of sugar are problematic for gestational diabetes.

(2) **Avoid artificial sweeteners:** Artificial sweeteners add sweetness to foods without adding calories. The FDA has approved Aspartame (Equal or NutraSweet), Rebaudioside A (Stevia), Acesulfame Potassium (Sunett), and Sucralose (Splenda) for use during pregnancy, however, the studies are now recommending that pregnant and lactating women should use these products with caution.[49] One Danish study shows an association between the

---

49   A. Sharma et al., "Artificial sweeteners as a sugar substitute: Are they really safe?" NCBI, May 2016, accessed September 24, 2017, https://www.ncbi.nlm.nih.gov/pmc/articles/PMC4899993/.

consumption of artificially sweetened beverages and preterm delivery.[50] Not to mention, studies are now suggesting that regular consumption of artificial sweeteners in the general population are actually associated with negative health outcomes such as type II diabetes and metabolic disorders, as opposed to helping to prevent them.[51]

③ **Reduce carbohydrate intake:** Carbohydrates are broken down to sugar by the digestive system and that sugar enters the blood. In response to this, blood sugar rises and insulin is released by the pancreas which prompts the sugar to be used as energy or to be stored in cells. Sometimes not enough insulin is created by the pancreas and that leads to high blood sugar levels as the sugar remains in the blood as opposed to getting used or stored. Carbohydrates affect blood sugar and insulin response more than proteins and fats so it is imperative to reduce carbohydrate intake if you suffer from gestational diabetes. I recommend an average of 150–175 grams of carbohydrates per day in general. You may need more or less based on your height, current weight, stage of pregnancy, age, and activity level.

④ **Obtain majority of carbohydrates from vegetables:** It is still important to eat carbohydrates during pregnancy—your primary carbohydrates should come from vegetable sources as they are low-glycemic. The Glycemic Index ranks carbohydrates in terms of how quickly they turn to sugar once digested. Most vegetables (notably green vegetables) are low-glycemic which means they raise blood sugar very minimally and slowly while providing energy, nutrients, and fiber.

⑤ **Eliminate carbohydrates from high-sugar fruits:** Like vegetables, low-glycemic fruits are another carbohydrate source that provide essential nutrients and antioxidants while resulting in marginal blood sugar increase and insulin response. Fruits such as avocado, tomato, and bell pepper are extremely low in carbohydrates and sugar so those can be a part of your gestational diabetes diet. Low-sugar

50　TI Halldorsson et al., "Intake of artificially sweetened soft drinks and risk of preterm delivery: a prospective cohort study in 59,334 Danish pregnant women.," NCBI, September 2010, accessed September 24, 2017, https://www.ncbi.nlm.nih.gov/pubmed/20592133.

51　S. Swithers, "Artificial sweeteners produce the counterintuitive effect of inducing metabolic derangements," NCBI, September 2013, accessed September 24, 2017, https://www.ncbi.nlm.nih.gov/pmc/articles/PMC3772345/.

fruits such as berries can be consumed in moderation (we recommend no more than one serving per day). High-glycemic fruits such as mango, figs, banana, and pineapple should be avoided as they cause spikes in the blood sugar and insulin response.

⑥ **Eat more proteins and healthy fats:** Protein and healthy fats have very little bearing on blood sugar so consuming more of these macronutrients (and less carbohydrates) is key to treating or preventing gestational diabetes. Protein and fats help to keep your blood sugar levels even and they assist with keeping your fuller for longer which may prevent spikes and drops in blood glucose. High-carbohydrate intake results in those spikes in blood sugar, followed by a "crash" which may lead to cravings for more carbohydrates. Keep in mind, it is critical to consume high-quality proteins and healthy fats (since not all proteins and fats are created equal). Wild salmon, organic meats/poultry, nuts, seeds, broccoli, spinach, quinoa, avocado, and extra-virgin olive oil are great examples of proteins and fats to consume, while items such as hot dogs, deli meats, fried foods, vegetable oil, and fast foods are best to be avoided.

⑦ **Do not eat any gluten-foods such as bread, pasta, crackers, and cereals (not even the whole wheat versions):** Gluten-containing foods such as bread, pasta, crackers, and cereals are high-glycemic—they will raise your blood sugar very quickly which triggers a substantial insulin response. During pregnancy, other hormones that are produced by the placenta impair insulin's ability to convert the sugar in the blood to the cells so assisting your body by not consuming these high-glycemic foods is extremely beneficial. The Glycemic Index ranks carbohydrate-containing foods with regard to how they are compared to sugar in terms of the rise in blood sugar they cause. Pure sugar is given a ranking of 100, meaning it will raise your blood sugar the most. Any item that receives a ranking of seventy or more is considered high-glycemic and should be eliminated. The average commercial white bread is given a glycemic index score of seventy-three whereas the average commercial wheat bread is given a score of sixty-nine. So yes, technically whole wheat bread is "better" than white bread but it is only marginally better and will still cause substantial rises in blood sugar as it is right on the border of being considered high-glycemic. For a reference point, carbohydrate sources such as broccoli, kale, cauliflower, tomato, Brussels sprouts, collard greens, and lettuces have Glycemic Index scores that are less than twenty.

⑧ **Do not eat gluten-free versions of bread, pasta, crackers, and cereals:** You may be wondering if the gluten-free versions of these foods are acceptable to consume while trying to manage or prevent gestational diabetes and the short answer is no. Gluten-free breads, pastas, crackers, and convenience foods are processed with replacement flours such as potato starch and tapioca starch. Unfortunately, these starches raise your blood sugar even more than typical gluten-containing wheat flours found in regular breads, pastas, and crackers. Even though these items are technically gluten-free, they are not *Whole Food Pregnancy* approved as they will only do a disservice to one who is trying to combat gestational diabetes and/or weight gain.

⑨ **Boil your sweet potatoes:** With some foods, the Glycemic Index can be confusing as preparation can actually alter the Glycemic Index ranking, and sweet potatoes fall under this category. Sweet potatoes are definitely a *Whole Food Pregnancy* food as they are loaded with nutrients such as vitamin A and beta-carotene, however, if you are treating or actively preventing gestational diabetes, please boil your sweet potato with the skin on—this will result in a low GI score of forty-six. If you bake your sweet potato for forty-five minutes, the composition and quality of the starches change, causing the score to jump to ninety-four which is considered very high and should be avoided, as high GI scores raise blood sugar the most!

⑩ **Eliminate sugary beverages:** Of course we all know that sodas should be eliminated, but there are still other beverages that are touted as being healthy but will worsen gestational diabetes. Sports drinks tend to be advertised as being a somewhat healthy alternative to sodas as they boast electrolytes, but these too are filled with sugars, additives, and artificial ingredients—the costs of these drinks definitely outweigh the benefits. There is much confusion about fruit juices in particular since we have always been taught that they are good to consume due to the vitamin content. In addition, it is a misconception that natural sugar coming from the fruit is unlike processed sugar in terms of the effect it has on our blood sugar, but the reality is that our bodies cannot distinguish between the fructose found in fruit from any other types of sugar. Water is the most beneficial beverage for pregnancy whether you have gestational diabetes or you are trying to prevent it.

(11) **Eat frequent small meals and snacks if you're hungry:** Eating frequently can help you stay full and fend off hunger or cravings. Incorporating protein and healthy fats in several small meals and snacks all day will help keep blood sugar levels even. If you are awake for sixteen hours per twenty-four day and you eat something every three hours, you will be eating around five to six times per day. Given you are consuming roughly 2200 calories per day, each small/meal snack will have an average of 400 calories.

Recommended Servings per Day for Gestational Diabetes

Food Category	Servings Per Day	Food Examples
Low-Glycemic Vegetables	5–8	Spinach, broccoli, kale, collard greens, cauliflower, cabbage, Brussels sprouts, bok choy, romaine lettuce, arugula
Low-Sugar Fruits	1–2	Tomato, bell pepper, olives, avocado, lemon, raspberries, strawberries, blueberries
Probiotic Foods	0–2	Greek yogurt (unsweetened), kefir (unsweetened), olives, sauerkraut, tempeh, natto
Starchy Produce	0–1	Sweet potato (boiled with skin on), fingerling potatoes (boiled with skin on), butternut squash, pumpkin
Protein	4–6	Wild Salmon, white fish, shellfish, chicken, eggs, turkey, grass-fed beef, spinach, broccoli, beans, lentils, quinoa, tempeh, natto
Healthy Fats	3–4	Walnuts, almonds, chia seeds, flaxseeds, extra-virgin olive oil, wild salmon, eggs, avocado
Caution Foods	0	Bread, pasta, cereal, crackers, fast food, fried foods, processed food, convenience meals, desserts

Contrary to the above *Whole Food Pregnancy* guidelines that help prevent or manage gestational diabetes, many doctors still promote meal plans for those with gestational diabetes that contain several daily servings of items such as whole wheat bread, whole wheat pasta, and cereals. As explained earlier in this chapter, these foods will only exacerbate the problem as they will greatly raise your blood sugar despite being whole wheat. So why do doctors still recommend these foods to combat gestational diabetes?

The United States food pyramid that was released in 1992 suggested eating six to eleven servings of grains every day so it has been engrained (no pun intended) in our society that we need hundreds of gluten-containing carbohydrates to be "healthy." Many medical professionals and nutritionists still base their recommendations on these trends despite the fact that it has been proven that large amounts of these high-glycemic carbohydrates will raise your blood sugar and may lead to gestational diabetes or type II diabetes. Yes, these recommendations have been revamped slightly; however, the new "MyPlate" still suggests that pregnant women eat eight slices of bread (or other equivalent grain-containing items) per day! The United States Department of Agriculture plays a heavy role in determining these guidelines and then these same guidelines are incorporated in nutrition education curriculum which is taught to nutritionists, as well as some doctors. Essentially, as opposed to being based on scientific research and evidence, these recommendations are influenced by food producers, manufacturers, and special interest groups. One of the USDA's largest priorities is to strengthen and support food, agriculture, and farming industries, so these guidelines may be disproportionately based on profit as opposed to the health of pregnant women and the rest of the general population.

I know it can be nerve-wracking to think of possible complications such as gestational diabetes and I definitely do not want to alarm you. I bring these issues up since they are becoming more common and the best way to combat them is with knowledge and preventative action. Good nutrition is a very powerful weapon to use through your whole pregnancy as it may greatly reduce the risk of pregnancy-related conditions.

Chapter 11
Growing Needs of the Second Trimester

Spanning from week thirteen to week twenty-seven, the second trimester is often referred to as the "honeymoon period," and I hope it is that way for you! If you suffered from morning sickness, that will hopefully be coming to an end now and you may even experience days of not feeling pregnant at all . . . well, until you feel your baby move for the first time, which will be unforgettable! According to the Institute of Medicine, if you are at a healthy weight, you will only need an average of 350 extra calories per day during the second trimester of your pregnancy. For example, if you were consuming an average of 1800 calories per day during the first trimester, you should now consume an average of 2150 calories per day during your second trimester. As we previously mentioned, you will see that I cover a wide range when it comes to calorie recommendations, considering a woman who is 4'11" tall and who weighed 95 pounds before conception will have different caloric needs than a woman who is 5'11" and weighed 170 pounds before conception.

When I mention calories, they are an average guideline to keep in mind, but remember that the types of calories are just as important (if not more)! If you stick to the recommended servings and proper portions found in Chapter 8, the calorie and nutrient intake will naturally fall into place. There are some specific nutrients that stand out as being especially beneficial during your second trimester of pregnancy and they are detailed below. The following nutrients have been vital during each trimester; however, they are superstars of this second trimester, so being mindful of adequate intake is especially important at this time.

Calcium

During the second trimester, your baby's bones and teeth are becoming denser, so your need for calcium remains double your requirement before pregnancy. If you do not consume enough calcium, your baby will draw from your own bones, which can lead to osteoporosis later on in life. According to the American Dietetic Association, pregnant women have the ability to absorb more calcium from food than usual as the body can sense the need from the developing fetus. Some sources of calcium are cooked kale, Greek yogurt, kefir, sardines with bones, canned salmon, broccoli, watercress, bok choy, okra, almonds, black-eyed peas, beans, and butternut squash.

Vitamin D

Vitamin D helps you absorb calcium, so while you are eating calcium-rich foods to assist with your baby's bone and teeth development, adequate amounts of vitamin D will help with your calcium stores, which will in turn help your baby's growth. Research also suggests that low maternal vitamin D is associated with unfavorable gestational outcomes such as preterm birth, gestational diabetes, and preeclampsia.[52] Vitamin D deficiency is prevalent worldwide, so it is imperative to get your levels checked and supplement accordingly. Some studies suggest that the current recommendation of 200–400 IUs of vitamin D for pregnant women is not sufficient and that supplementing daily with 1000–6400 IUs of vitamin D would help to alleviate deficiency without toxicity.[53] Some sources of vitamin D are responsible sun exposure, fatty fish, eggs, and beef liver.

Magnesium

Magnesium is the third needed party with vitamin D and calcium. Magnesium helps you metabolize vitamin D, which in turn helps you absorb calcium. Since your baby's skeletal system is rapidly growing and forming, she can use all the help she can get and magnesium will provide great benefit to the other second trimester superstar nutrients, calcium and vitamin D. Some examples of magnesium sources are spinach, chard, pumpkin seeds, Greek yogurt, kefir, almonds, black beans, avocado, and dark chocolate.

---

52 SQ Wei, "Vitamin D and pregnancy outcomes.," NCBI, December 2014, accessed September 27, 2017, https://www.ncbi. nlm.nih.gov/pubmed/25310531.

53 Samar Al Emadi and Mohammed Hammoudeh, "Vitamin D study in pregnant women and their babies," NCBI, November 01, 2013, accessed August 30, 2017, https://www.ncbi.nlm.nih.gov/pmc/articles/PMC3991049/.

Iron

Your need for iron is especially great during the second trimester, and yet around half of all pregnant women do not get adequate amounts. Your blood volume is increasing at a rapid rate and you need sufficient iron to create hemoglobin, which is a protein in red blood cells. Iron also helps to transport oxygen from your lungs to your baby, as well as the rest of your body. Some sources of iron are red meat, poultry, oily fish, shellfish, beans, lentils, raisins, and green leafy vegetables.

In addition to the above-mentioned nutrients, it is vital that you are gaining weight at this time. If you were considered to be at normal weight before pregnancy, you can expect to gain an average of one to two pounds per week during your second trimester. It can be counterintuitive for some to be happy about that number rising on the scale each week but yes, be happy! That rising number means your baby is growing beautifully and your body is too, in preparation for your little one. According to the American Pregnancy Association, your weight gain (by the end of pregnancy) will be distributed according to this chart.

	Average Weight
Baby	7.5 pounds
Placenta	1.5 pounds
Increased Fluids	4 pounds
Uterus	2 pounds
Breast Tissue	2 pounds
Increased Blood Volume	4 pounds
Maternal Stores (fat, protein, nutrients)	7 pounds
Amniotic Fluid	2 pounds
Total Weight Gain	30 pounds

Although it is critical to gain weight during pregnancy, it is just as important to avoid excessive weight gain due to improper food consumption—quite the balancing act! The foods recommended throughout *The Whole Food Pregnancy Plan* are designed to give the most bang for the buck with regard to nutrients per calorie/kilocalorie. Of course you will have cravings and there is some wiggle room for those cravings in the 90/10 cheat rule (allowing 10 percent of your total calorie intake to be allotted to your cheat foods of choice); however, it is advised to strictly limit empty-calorie foods if possible. Regular consumption of these empty calorie foods can lead to excessive weight gain and gestational diabetes, and can implicate the health of your unborn baby.

Not to mention, several of the foods we are about to discuss have harmful additives and preservatives that are not ideal to consume, whether you are expecting a baby or not.

Genetically Modified Organisms (GMO)

Some crops in our food supply are genetically modified in order to be able to withstand being sprayed by Roundup, which is a weed killer that contains glyphosate. Glyphosate, the most widely-used herbicide in the world, has been categorized as a "probable human carcinogen" by the World Health Organization. Non-organic soy, corn, and a variety of other crops have been genetically altered to tolerate direct spraying of the herbicide, and items like wheat are also treated with glyphosate containing Roundup right before harvest, resulting in grain/gluten-based food products left with a glyphosate residue.

There are some concerns that glyphosate could be correlated with pregnancy-related issues. A recent study has shown that levels of glyphosate found in expectant mothers' bodily fluids were correlated with birth outcomes that were unfavorable. Urine samples were taken from pregnant women and it was found that significantly shorter pregnancies with lower birth weights were correlated with higher glyphosate levels found in the pregnant mothers' urine samples. Research shows that preterm birth is associated with lower cognitive ability as well as developing diabetes, high blood pressure, and heart disease later in life.[54] To avoid GMO foods, look for products labeled as "certified organic" as these items are not allowed to contain genetically modified organisms. Moreover, produce is labeled with PLU (price look-up) codes which are located on the sticker, found on the piece of produce. To guarantee you are not buying a genetically modified food that is likely to have been treated with glyphosate, choose the codes that begin with the number nine—this means the food is organic!

Fast Food and Processed Foods

Yes, there is a general consensus that fast food and processed foods can be detrimental to one's health, but the general

---

54 Paul Winchester, Cathy Proctor, and Jun Ying, "County-level pesticide use and risk of shortened gestation and preterm birth, "NCBI, November 23, 2015, accessed September 01, 2017, https://www.ncbi.nlm.nih.gov/pmc/articles/PMC5067698/pdf/APA-105-e107.pdf.

blanket statement that they are "bad" still may not convince you to steer clear of them during pregnancy, so we will explore some popular fast food and commercially prepared food ingredients below. In fact, eight in ten Americans say they eat fast food at least once per month and five in ten admit to consuming fast food at least once per week. By the second trimester, your baby can actually begin to taste the foods you are eating and this causes your baby to become familiar with particular foods.[55] Training your baby's taste buds to enjoy fast foods, processed foods, and their harmful ingredients may put your child on a path of unhealthy food choices before she is even born. Not to mention, some studies suggest that regular fast food consumption can have negative effects (such as asthma) on your unborn baby's health.[56]

Fast food meals and commercially packaged foods are known to be loaded with empty calories, high-glycemic carbohydrates, sugar, and bad fats, but that is just the tip of the iceberg. If you order the typical burger, fries, and a soft drink at a fast food establishment, you are likely to consume a combination of trans-fatty acids, Butylated Hydroxyanisole, hydrolyzed vegetable proteins, and artificial dyes and flavors. You do not want to transfer these ingredients to your developing baby, and even if one is not pregnant, fast food and processed foods are best eliminated due to their content. Let's take a look at these ingredients below.

Butylated Hydroxyanisole

Butylated Hydroxyanisole (BHA) is a chemical food additive put in oils so the oils can be used multiple times without going rancid. BHA is a known carcinogen and several studies have shown links between the chemical and cancerous tumors in animals, and stomach cancer in humans. Many fast food baked goods, fried foods, dehydrated potatoes, and meat products contain butylated hydroxyanisole.

Trans-Fatty Acids

Trans-fatty acids (or trans fats) are created by adding hydrogen to vegetable oil and many fast food establishments use this type of fat because it is cheap and has a

---

55   Jennifer Savage, Jennifer Orlet Fisher, and Leann Birch, "Parental Influence on Eating Behavior," NCBI, March 02, 2007, accessed September 01, 2017, https://www.ncbi.nlm.nih.gov/pmc/articles/PMC2531152/.

56   OS Von Ehrenstein et al., "Fast food consumption in pregnancy and subsequent asthma symptoms in young children.," NCBI, September 26, 2015, accessed September 01, 2017, https://www.ncbi.nlm.nih.gov/pubmed/26109272.

longer shelf life than other fats. When this type of oil is used in deep fryers, it doesn't have to be changed as often since it takes longer to spoil. Trans fats are known for raising your LDL (bad) cholesterol while lowering your HDL (good) cholesterol, but there are also detrimental effects from trans fats on your unborn baby. Animal studies have shown that regular consumption of trans-fatty acids has led to memory difficulties, amplified emotional reactions, and oxidative injury in the brain cells of babies.[57]

Hydrolyzed Vegetable Proteins

Vegetable protein—it doesn't sound so bad. Hydrolyzed vegetable proteins are created when foods such as soy, corn, and wheat are boiled in hydrochloric acid and neutralized with sodium hydroxide which breaks the proteins in the vegetables down into amino acids. Monosodium glutamate (MSG) is one of the amino acids; MSG is regarded as "safe" in moderation by many popular pregnancy websites and sources. However, animal studies have shown that MSG does cross the placenta and may have negative effects on the memory of the fetus and long-term ability to learn.[58]

Dyes and Artificial Flavors

Dyes and artificial flavors are used by many fast food establishments and commercial food manufacturers to replace real food by providing fake color and flavor to menu items. Brightly colored desserts, sodas, and macaroni and cheese contain dyes that are possible carcinogens, such as Yellow No. 5 and No. 6. Some countries, including England, require labeling of products that contain Yellow No. 5 and No. 6 as they have been linked to hyperactivity in children. The United States has banned some dyes, though Blue No. 1, Blue No. 2, Green No. 3, Red No. 3, Red No. 40, Yellow No. 5, and Yellow No. 6 still remain on the FDA's approved list—yet another reason to check your ingredients labels!

---

57 CS Pase et al., "Influence of perinatal trans fat on behavioral responses and brain oxidative status of adolescent rats acutely exposed to stress," NCBI, September 05, 2013, accessed September 02, 2017, https://www.ncbi.nlm.nih.gov/pubmed/23742847.

58 J. Gao et al., "[Transplacental neurotoxic effects of monosodium glutamate on structures and functions of specific brain areas of filial mice]," NCBI, February 01, 1994, accessed September 02, 2017, https://www.ncbi.nlm.nih.gov/pubmed/8085168.

Dimethylpolysiloxane

Dimethylpolysiloxane is derived from silicon and is found in hair and skin conditioners, cosmetics, and Silly Putty. It is used in cooking oils as an anti-foaming agent to prevent spattering oil, and is found in items like chicken nuggets, French fries, and fried sandwiches. In addition, it even lurks in fountain drinks to limit the excess foam you typically get with canned and bottled sodas. Dimethylpolysiloxane is used in a wide variety of fast food establishments including ones that claim to use higher quality, healthier, and even organic ingredients.

Azodicarbonamide

One of the more recently controversial food additives, as it is used in yoga mats, azodicarbonamide (ADA) is a flour bleaching agent and dough conditioner that is banned across most of Europe, Australia, and Singapore. Considered to be a carcinogen, ADA is linked to cancer, neurological disorders, cell mutations, and disrupted hormone functions in animals. Many fast food and commercial food manufacturers have eliminated this ingredient from their products, but it remains in a variety of processed foods.

Making the best food choices for you and your baby throughout your whole pregnancy can be hard sometimes—especially when there are so many hidden ingredients in our food supply! I will admit that I, too, occasionally craved a fast food burger, fries, and soda, but I just tried to remind myself that everything I put in my body, I was putting into my baby's body as well. No one is perfect, so if you slip up here and there, don't be hard on yourself, but if possible ,please avoid regular consumption of these dangerous foods. Pregnancy is only temporary and you're almost there—your healthy lifestyle and the health of your baby will all be worth it.

Chapter 12
Welcome to the Third Trimester

You're almost ready to meet your little one! Your third trimester goes from week twenty-eight to week forty and during this time, your baby is growing rapidly so sticking to your healthy food regimen from trimesters one and two is very important. You can still follow the food plan that was outlined in Chapter 8—simply add some calories (around an average of 450 calories more than what you ate before pregnancy) to your daily intake as your little one will need an extra boost at this time.

As always, the types of calories are just as important (if not more) than the amounts of calories consumed. There are some specific nutrients that stand out as being especially beneficial during your final trimester of pregnancy, and they are detailed below. The following nutrients have been vital during each trimester; however, they are superstars of this third trimester, so being mindful of adequate intake is critical.

Iron

Your blood volume is still increasing, so consuming an ample amount of iron is critical in order to build enough healthy red blood cells since hemoglobin (found in red blood cells) carries oxygen throughout your body. Being low on iron is common during the third trimester since your baby takes iron from you for his/her own stores. Not getting enough iron can result in anemia, premature delivery, and low birth weight.[59] Iron can be found in red meat, poultry, oily fish, shellfish, beans, lentils, raisins, and green leafy vegetables.

Protein

Your baby is doing a lot of growing in this trimester and protein has amino acids which help his/her muscles and tissues to grow strong and healthy. Coincidentally, many protein sources also contain iron as well as zinc, which is associated with

---

59 TO Scholl, "Iron status during pregnancy: setting the stage for mother and infant.," NCBI, May 2005, accessed September 29, 2017, https://www.ncbi.nlm.nih.gov/pubmed/15883455.

the production of enzymes and insulin.[60] Also, enough protein helps to maintain even blood sugar levels which can prevent gestational diabetes and cravings. Protein can be found in meat, poultry, seafood, beans, lentils, peas, quinoa, broccoli, kale, spinach, nuts, and seeds.

Vitamin B6

Vitamin B6 (also called pyridoxine) helps to convert food into energy. Vitamin B6 will help you metabolize the extra protein you're taking in to assist with your baby's muscle and tissue development.[61] Meanwhile, B6 also assists with the maintenance of healthy potassium and sodium levels. Vitamin B6 can be found in sunflower seeds, pistachio nuts, flaxseeds, walnuts, hazelnuts, wild salmon, halibut, turkey, chicken, pork chops, dried prunes, dried apricots, raisins, lean beef, banana, avocado, and cooked spinach.

Calcium

Remember how your baby was lightly fluttering last trimester? Those little flutters have now probably turned into the occasional sharp jab or kick! Your baby's bones are really developing now and becoming denser, resulting in the increased need for calcium. Your baby will draw calcium directly from your own bones and teeth, so it's vital to consume enough for your baby to use so your own does not get depleted. Calcium can be found in salmon, sardines, Greek yogurt, kefir, spinach, kale, collard greens, white beans, dried figs, oranges, almonds, and oatmeal.

Magnesium

Magnesium is calcium's sidekick! Magnesium helps you absorb calcium, as well as building and repairing body tissues. This mineral also eases leg cramps, relaxes muscles, and some studies show that it may assist with preterm labor prevention.[62] Magnesium can be found in artichokes, pumpkin seeds, almonds, black beans, dark leafy greens, avocados, bananas, and fish.

---

60 AB Chausmer, "Zinc, insulin and diabetes.," NCBI, April 1998, accessed September 29, 2017, https://www.ncbi.nlm.nih.gov/pubmed/9550453.

61 Bender, DA. "Vitamin B6 requirements and recommendations." NCBI. May 1989. Accessed September 29, 2017. https://www.ncbi.nlm.nih.gov/pubmed/2661220.

62 J Durlach, "New data on the importance of gestational Mg deficiency.," NCBI, December 2004, accessed September 29, 2017, https://www.ncbi.nlm.nih.gov/pubmed/15637217.

Choline

Choline promotes the proper functioning of cells, and since your baby is growing rapidly in this trimester, choline is key. The Journal of American College of Nutrition has reported that choline may be depleted during pregnancy, so consuming adequate choline will assist with keeping your levels in proper range. Choline is vital for your baby's memory development and can be found in eggs, shrimp, scallops, chicken, turkey, cod, salmon, collard greens, cauliflower, cabbage, broccoli, garbanzo beans, and lentils.

Healthy Fats

Your baby's brain is developing at an exponential rate, and omega-3 fatty acids (specifically docosahexaenoic acid or DHA) will help to facilitate this growth. In fact, adequate DHA consumption has been linked to improved infant cognition as well as the formation of your baby's nervous system, according to numerous studies.[63] Some research also suggests that maternal omega-3 fatty acid consumption is associated with lower risk of postpartum depression.[64] In addition, building your own healthy fat stores will help to prepare you for breastfeeding (if you choose to do so) and provide energy for labor. Healthy fats can be found in wild salmon, avocado, nuts, seeds, grass-fed beef, and egg yolks.

Vitamins D3 and K2

Fat-soluble vitamins D3 and K2 are extremely valuable for bone health. Vitamin D3 is now widely acknowledged for its importance; however, K2 isn't quite as commonly known for assisting with healthy bones and tissues. Some sources of D3 are wild salmon, herring, sardines, egg yolks, fish oil, and responsible sun exposure. K2 can be found in fermented foods such as sauerkraut and natto, and organ meats (liver, kidney, heart, tongue, etc.).

Unfortunately, there are some common third trimester nutritional issues so if you face any or all of the following, not to worry—there are ways to combat them! As I discussed earlier in this chapter, low iron or even anemia can occur in the third trimester, so make sure you're eating your iron.

---

63 NL Morse, "Benefits of Docosahexaenoic Acid, Folic Acid, Vitamin D and Iodine on Foetal and Infant Brain Development and Function Following Maternal Supplementation during Pregnancy and Lactation," NCBI, July 2017, accessed September 29, 2017, https://www.ncbi.nlm.nih.gov/pmc/articles/PMC3407995/.

64 J. Wojcicki and MB Heyman, "Maternal omega-3 fatty acid supplementation and risk for perinatal maternal depression," NCBI, May 2011, accessed September 29, 2017, https://www.ncbi.nlm.nih.gov/pmc/articles/PMC3119925/.

In addition to proper medical care and nutrition, it is essential for expectant mothers to be educated and to be provided with information regarding postpartum depression (PPD). Postpartum depression is a severe form of depression which can occur after delivery that interferes with a new mother's mood and her ability to function in daily life. It is not uncommon for women to report that they were unaware of the signs or symptoms of this disorder. Symptoms may often go ignored, as new mothers may attribute them to simply being tired due to lack of sleep as a result of caring for her newborn. Oftentimes, women may experience embarrassment or shame, which can prevent them from sharing their symptoms and feelings with others. Symptoms of PPD include sleep and eating disturbances, anxiety, extreme sadness, and severe fatigue or exhaustion.[65] Additional and more severe symptoms can include excessive anger, irritability, feelings of worthlessness, disinterest in Baby, fear of not being a good mother or of being left alone with the infant, and even suicidal thoughts.[66] It is important that pregnant women as well as relatives and close friends are educated about the signs and symptoms of the disorder, so that treatment can be provided as soon as possible to enable the best opportunity for recovery. A woman who is diligent in taking care of herself both physically and mentally will be in much better "shape" should she develop postpartum depression following the birth of her new baby. While there are many causes of postpartum depression, research suggests that it is more common for women with deficiencies in several essential minerals and nutrients to experience depression.[67] Also, studies have concluded that those with higher intakes of nutritious foods such as vegetables, fruit, and fish tend to have a decreased likelihood of experiencing depression or depressive symptoms.[68] When a woman believes that she may have postpartum depression or has taken notice that even one or two symptoms are present, it is crucial that she seek medical and mental health attention immediately as treatment for the condition is necessary in order to ensure the health and well-being for mother, baby, and family members.

—Kara Cruz, MA, Registered Associate Marriage and Family Therapist

65 "Postpartum Depression Facts," National Institute of Mental Health, accessed September 10, 2017, https://www.nimh.nih.gov/health/publications/postpartum-depression-facts/index.shtml.

66 American Psychological Association, "What is postpartum depression and anxiety?" accessed September 11, 2017 from http://www.apa.org/pi/women/resources/reports/postpartum-depression.aspx.

67 Lisa M. Bodnar and Katherine L. Wisner, "Nutrition and Depression: Implications for Improving Mental Health Among Childbearing-Aged Women," Biological psychiatry, November 01, 2005, accessed September 13, 2017, https://www.ncbi.nlm.nih.gov/pmc/articles/PMC4288963/.

68 Adrienne O'Neil et al., "Preventing mental health problems in offspring by targeting dietary intake of pregnant women," BMC Medicine, November 14, 2014, accessed September 13, 2017, https://bmcmedicine.biomedcentral.com/articles/10.1186/s12916-014-0208-0.

If you suffer from heartburn, eat smaller meals and avoid spicy foods. Eating papaya is a natural remedy for fighting heartburn, but make sure it is ripe, as unripe papaya contains pepsin which can cause contractions and early labor. If you're facing fatigue, try to avoid sweet foods as those foods will lead to sharp increases and decreases in blood sugar—that blood sugar crash will add unwanted fatigue. Increased urination certainly comes with the territory of the third trimester, but it's a temporary inconvenience so still drink plenty of water. To relieve or avoid constipation, eat plenty of gluten-free fiber sources such as raspberries, artichoke, lentils, peas, beans, and leafy greens. Swelling is another common issue that occurs in the third trimester—drinking plenty of water will help, since water intake flushes the body and actually reduces water retention; eating foods low in sodium and high in potassium such as sweet potato, yogurt, and banana will fight swelling. I certainly hope you aren't experiencing many of these issues but even if you are, you're in the home stretch of your pregnancy journey, so hang in there!

Being in the home stretch of your pregnancy means that you are probably thinking about labor and delivery and the vast amount of decisions that need to be made for this process. If your goal is to give birth vaginally, you may want to consider eating during labor. It is likely that you have been told that you should not eat or even that you will not be allowed to eat during your labor, however, many current studies state there is no harm involved in low-risk women eating during labor.[69]

Women have been advised to fast during labor due to the extremely minimal risk of aspiration, resulting from inhaling recently eaten food into the lungs while unconscious, under general anesthesia during a Cesarean section (this recommendation was founded based on studies conducted in the 1940s, however, this frame of thought may be unwarranted based on today's practices).[70] Nowadays, most C-sections are not performed using general anesthesia—epidurals and spinal injections are used for the majority of C-sections, meaning you will be conscious during

69   M. Singata, J. Tranmer, and G. Gyte, "Eating and drinking in labour," NCBI, August 22, 2013, accessed September 29, 2017, https://www.ncbi.nlm.nih.gov/pubmedhealth/PMH0012411/.

70   JD Sperling, JD Dahlke, and BM Sibai, "Restriction of oral intake during labor: whither are we bound?" NCBI, May 2016, , accessed September 29, 2017, https://www.ncbi.nlm.nih.gov/pubmed/26812080.

the surgery. If the case arises where you are unconscious for a C-section, the anesthetist gently compresses the esophagus which prevents possible inhalation of anything from your stomach. Due to improvements in anesthesia, it is very rare that aspiration occurs in laboring women; however, if you are definitely planning a C-section, you will probably be advised to not eat at least six to eight hours before your operation and it is important to respect your care provider's policy on this matter.

Since I had no known issues with my own health or my baby's that would warrant a scheduled C-section, I chose to eat during labor as my goal was to give birth vaginally and I wanted as much energy as possible. The caloric and energy demands of labor are comparable to running a marathon and if those caloric demands are not met, your body will turn to fat for energy, which can lessen contractions and delay labor. Not to mention, fatigue can set in during long labors and lack of strength and energy due to lack of calories can lead to the inability to push the baby out after several hours of labor. If you are high-risk due to issues such as gestational diabetes, preeclampsia, and obesity, it may be safest to withhold foods

during labor; please consult your physician if you have questions.

Before making the personal decision to eat during labor, I did consult with my doula, who has coached more than 250 births. She explained that I would need the stored calories for what would be the longest workout of my life and she was absolutely correct. With that being said, I believe that my food intake during labor was one of the key strategies that got me through my twenty-hour birthing "workout." As in any other sporting event, if I hadn't fueled up properly, I probably wouldn't have finished successfully.

Here's what I ate and drank:

7:00 a.m. (start of labor)—water
8:00 a.m.—two eggs and a banana
10:00 a.m.—more water
1:00 p.m.—half of a salad with grilled chicken, avocado, tomato, onion, beets, and pine nuts; more water
2:00 p.m.—more water
5:00 p.m.—the other half of the chicken salad
7:00 p.m. (admitted to hospital)—nothing
9:00 p.m.—nothing
12:00 a.m.—nothing
3:06 a.m.—end of labor!

During active labor, the last thing on my mind was eating—thankfully, the chicken salad I finished at five o'clock fueled me enough to get me through to when my baby was born at 3:06 a.m.! I, personally, found eating during labor to be extremely beneficial, and some studies are finding the same, as even the World Health Organization states that laboring women should not be restricted from eating and drinking liquids.[71] If you do choose to eat during labor (after consulting with your health care providers), many sources suggest consuming very small snacks, since digestion is slowed down during labor.

When all was said and done, I was absolutely famished despite the fact that I had eaten much more than the typical laboring woman. Like participating in any other high-intensity event that will be long in duration, burning a few thousand calories, fueling up is what worked for me. Whether to eat or not during labor should be considered on a case-by-case basis as what may be risky for one may be perfectly safe for another, so as always, consult your physician, midwife, or doula to see what may be best for you.

Some examples of labor foods/beverages I recommend are:

Light soups, fruits, applesauce, fresh smoothies, raw nuts/seeds, nut butters, yogurt, quinoa, oatmeal, eggs, water, tea, ice chips, ice cubes made with honey-sweetened tea

---

71 NC Sharts-Hopko, "Oral intake during labor: a review of the evidence.," NCBI, July 2010, , accessed September 29, 2017, https://www.ncbi.nlm.nih.gov/pubmed/20585208.

Chapter 13
The Fourth Trimester– Postpartum Weight Loss

First of all, congratulations on the new addition to your family! As you know, the initial days and weeks (and sometimes months) of motherhood can be quite an adjustment, so do not feel pressured to put this chapter into action immediately and always consult with your doctor regarding postpartum weight loss. The following nutrition principles and guidelines are recommended for nursing and non-nursing mothers, though I do provide special instructions for nursing mothers in the following chapter.

The tactics to use to lose the baby weight will be extremely similar whether you are nursing or not. The primary difference is that nursing mothers will require some additional calories that non-nursing mothers do not require since milk production and breastfeeding does burn calories. The number of extra calories the nursing mother requires depends on factors such as age, activity level, maternal fat stores, and how often she is nursing. One may require as little as 200 extra calories per day or as much as 500 extra calories per day. A good rule of thumb to follow (whether you're breast-feeding or not) is to listen to your body and eat consciously. Eating consciously means eating when you are hungry and stopping when you are 80 percent full. It is easier said than done sometimes, but when we eat consciously, we avoid eating out of boredom, stress, or social pressure. Also, it is best to focus on your food instead of allocating attention to a book or movie since many tend to overeat while their minds are occupied by something else. During my personal postpartum weight loss journey (as well as my pregnancy), I never counted calories but I always kept this "Seven Scales of Hunger" chart in mind before I ate and while I was eating, and I always tried to remain around level four.

Seven Scales of Hunger

7. **About to burst:** Ate way too much food, but it was fun! Same feeling you may experience after Thanksgiving dinner or a birthday party and you think you may never want to see food again.

6. **Extremely full:** Feeling some discomfort/bloat and need to lie down.

5. **Pretty full:** Had a few extra bites after being satiated and won't need to eat again for some time.

4. **Comfortably satisfied:** Ate for fullness and not for sport; stopped when 80 percent full (this is easiest to attain when you eat slowly so your brain has time to signal to your stomach).

3. **A tad bit uncomfortable:** Didn't eat quite enough (around 70 percent full) and feel a snack (or more) is needed in the near future.

2. **Uncomfortable:** May have the "growling" sensation in the stomach and/or experience low energy.

1. **Miserable:** Extremely low on energy, unable to focus on tasks, and possibly irritable.

Just remember that one of the primary ways to lose the baby weight is to keep portions and caloric intake in proper range. Since I don't want to hold you to counting calories and weighing food (you are officially way too busy for that now!), I want to emphasize mindful eating, so the use of the above scale is very beneficial. Other postpartum weight loss principles I would like to discuss are below.

Principle ① Almost Everything Counts

Little decisions we make every day add up to create a significant long-term result. One may argue that a soda with lunch will not cause diabetes or significant weight gain and that's correct—one soda will not do that. The problem is that one soda at lunch potentially turns into thirty sodas per month. Thirty sodas per month equal 278 teaspoons of pure sugar. Sugar turns into fat once digested. Occasional splurges are realistic but they have to be occasional and the portion size should be controlled. The "this one soda will not kill me" attitude may be detrimental if that train of thought is repeated over and over again.

If you maintain a consistently healthy diet, don't feel bad about splurging once in a while. A large piece of cake at a birthday party is just fine—as long as you haven't had other servings of junk food that week. The most difficult aspect of this principle is being honest with yourself. If you feel as if you are not losing the baby weight quickly enough, try jotting down all of your food for a couple of days to see where some of the red flags may be occurring. Also, if you're someone who is still having some cravings (possibly due to nursing), keep the 90/10 cheat rule in mind—10 percent of your total caloric intake can be dedicated to cheats foods, which amounts to an average of 200 calories per day.

Principle ② Eliminate Bread, Pasta, Crackers, Cereal

I definitely recommend that you eat carbohydrates, but not these! We find our carbohydrates in items such as green vegetables, low sugar fruits, quinoa, and lentils. Gluten-containing foods such as bread, pasta, cereal, and crackers are high on the Glycemic Index—that means they convert into sugar quickly once they digest; that sugar then turns into fat if not burned off.

As previously discussed (see page 82), wheat bread, whole grain cereals, and whole wheat pastas are essentially

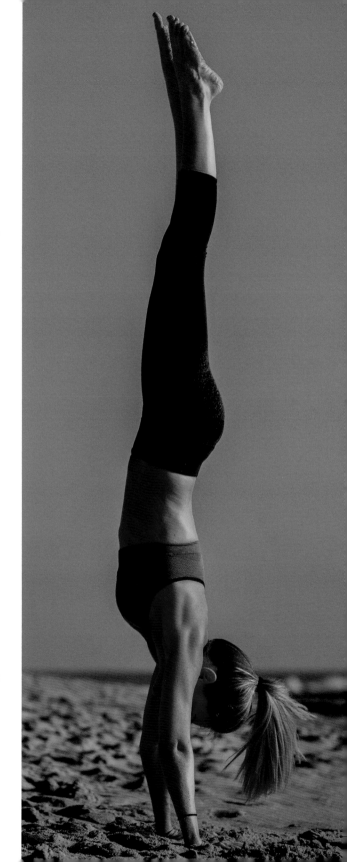

the same products as white bread, white crackers, and white pasta. The only major difference is that the wheat/brown options have a little bit more fiber (that's the brown coloring). For example, a piece of white bread has a ranking of 73 on the Glycemic Index and a piece of wheat bread has a ranking of 69. The Glycemic Index measures how quickly certain foods turn into sugar once digested—anything over 55 is considered high or bad. So yes, the wheat bread is slightly better than white but it still converts to sugar quickly, resulting in raised blood sugar levels and fat storage. If you are looking for fiber, artichokes, raspberries, almonds, broccoli, pears, apples, and turnip greens have just as much fiber if not more than wheat bread, whole grain crackers, and whole wheat pasta.

Principle ③ You Do Not "Need" Bread and Pasta to be Healthy

People do need to consume carbohydrates to be healthy but what many don't realize is that carbohydrates are found in several foods—not just the obvious gluten-containing items such as bread, pasta, crackers, and cereals. The not-so-obvious carbohydrates are consumed regularly and they do add up quickly.

Not eliminating or severely limiting your intake of bread, pasta, crackers, and cereals may possibly create an abundance of unused carbohydrates which will convert into sugar and then into fat. Some examples of not-so-obvious carbohydrate-containing foods are: 1 apple (21g), carrots (10 baby size=10g), yogurt (½ cup=5g), raw almonds (serving=8g), oatmeal (¼ cup=27g), and cooked peas (½ cup=8g). If one eats several servings of gluten-containing foods per day in addition to all of the hidden/not-so-obvious carbohydrates in other foods, weight loss could be extremely difficult.

Principle ④ Control Calories and Portions

Many people eat far more calories than their bodies need. Despite the fact that the main purpose of food is to fuel our bodies, it is commonly used for comfort, fun, social purposes, and a solution to boredom. Eating proper portions and not until you feel "stuffed" is a key component to achieving and maintaining your ideal weight.

The average American is told to consume 2,000 calories per day, but this figure is completely wrong for millions of people. For example, if you are a woman who is 5'4" and want to weigh 125 pounds., your required intake will range anywhere from 1400–1900 calories per day depending on age, activity level, whether or not you are nursing, and the frequency of your nursing.

Principle ⑤ Eat Nutrient-Dense Foods

It is imperative to keep portions and caloric intake in proper ranges, but a factor that is just as important (if not more) is making sure those calories are nutrient-dense. Eating 1800 calories of pizza, ice cream, and soda per day is extremely different than eating 1800 calories of green veggies, eggs, fish, low sugar fruits, and oatmeal per day. Choosing foods low in nutrients is very dangerous and may lead to vitamin, mineral, and nutrient deficiency in your breast milk as well as in your own body, which is linked to a host of health problems such as fatigue, osteoporosis, and even cancer. Moreover, when one eats a regular diet of empty calories and junk food, the body will have constant cravings as it's searching for the nutrients it needs. Some of my favorite healthy, postpartum weight loss foods are green veggies, low sugar fruits (raspberries, tomato, avocado, blueberries, strawberries, apples, blackberries), lean proteins (fish, chicken, grass fed beef, turkey), beans and legumes, quinoa, oatmeal, and good fats (avocado, salmon, raw nuts and seeds, extra-virgin olive oil, eggs).

Principle ⑥ Avoid Sugar

The average American eats 88 grams of sugar per day—that's 22 teaspoons! The recommended daily allowance of sugar is 30 grams for women and 45 grams for men. Too much sugar is dangerous because if you don't burn it, it can store as fat. Also, when products containing sugar (or products which convert to sugar) are consumed, the blood sugar rises, resulting in the need for the pancreas to release insulin. If you make your pancreas do too much work with regard to releasing large amounts of insulin throughout the day to control blood sugar levels, Type II Diabetes may result. Not to mention, the spikes in blood sugar and then the low which occurs soon after will cause constant cravings for food, so it's a vicious cycle!

There are many hidden sugar sources in the grocery store; many carbohydrate sources are high-glycemic and will convert to sugar almost as quickly as pure sugar does, and more often than not these products contain gluten. Some examples of hidden sugar sources are bread (wheat and white), crackers, bagels, pasta, and boxed cereals. To keep your blood sugar levels even, focus on low-glycemic carbohydrates (green vegetables, low sugar fruits, beans, legumes, Greek yogurt, oatmeal, and quinoa), lean proteins, and good fats.

Principle ⑦ Grocery List

Before leaving for the grocery store, make a list of nutritious foods and stick to it. If you don't buy junk food and have it around the house, you are much less likely to eat junk food. For recommended grocery items, please see the list in Chapter 3.

Principle ⑧ Eliminate or Limit Junk and Fast Food

Thousands of unhealthy, fattening, and dangerous food items have become "normal" and mainstream. A lot of these danger foods have become so socially acceptable that it can be thought of as strange to not participate in the consumption. It is critical to your weight management that these items be regarded as treats or special occasions—not typical, everyday food. Of course everyone is entitled to a splurge here and there but it is imperative to severely limit servings of junk food items such as fast food, pizza, soda, candy, cookies, cake, donuts, fried foods, and ice cream.

Principle ⑨ Be Prepared at Work

The workplace is, typically, a junk food haven. Office donuts, cookies, chips, sodas, and candy vending machines are incredibly tempting, especially when you're hungry. Not to mention, unhealthy snacking may be the majority in your office, so the "everybody's doing it" attitude adds to the temptation of giving in. Not being hungry can be the most effective way of combating the weight-gaining food that's in your workplace. It only takes five minutes to put together a healthy snack pack that will keep your hunger satiated and blood sugar levels even. It's as easy as putting a few healthy snacks in a bag the night before work—items like hardboiled eggs, raw nuts, vegetables and hummus, Greek yogurt, low sugar fruits, and healthy dinner leftovers.

Principle ⑩ Healthy Restaurant Choices

You can still lose the baby weight while dining out! If you're one who has a hectic work schedule or you just enjoy eating in restaurants, it is still realistic to bounce back to your pre-pregnancy weight in no time. Try to employ these key concepts when eating in restaurants:

- Skip the bread basket—even if it's put in front of you, kindly ask the server to take it away.
- Replace rice and pasta side dishes with vegetables.
- Use oil and vinegar for salad dressing.
- Eliminate bread dishes (i.e., sandwiches and burgers); if you order a sandwich or burger, ask your server to wrap it in lettuce (most restaurants will oblige).
- Avoid soup—it's usually full of sodium, bad oils, thickeners, and other weight-gaining ingredients.
- Ask for sauce on the side.
- Order fresh fruit or berries for dessert.
- Avoid waffles, French toast, pancakes, donuts, pastries, or hash browns at breakfast.

- If a restaurant meal is huge (and they usually are), take half of it home and have it for lunch the next day.
- National restaurant chains are required to have nutrition information on site. Check it out—it may save you a thousand calories!

Principle ⑪ Don't Drink Your Calories

A fruit juice with breakfast, Starbucks Frappuccino in the afternoon, and one soda at dinner add up to almost 900 calories and 100 grams of sugar! People can tend to ignore liquid calories and don't realize how easily they compile and result in weight gain. The habit of drinking water is a key staple to losing the baby weight. Unfortunately, soda and fruit juice have around the same amounts of calories, carbohydrates, and sugar. Even though fruit juice has natural sugar, it's still sugar and sugar turns into fat if it isn't burned. If you're looking for a good source of Vitamin C without the added sugar, opt for items like broccoli, Brussels sprouts, or raspberries.

Principle (12) Step Off the Wagon–Don't Fall

If you maintain balanced nutrition on a regular basis then splurging occasionally will not hurt your postpartum weight loss as long as you return to your good habits immediately after the splurge. Also, if you plan your splurges ahead of time, you will be nutritionally prepared to afford your treat. If you know you're going to a restaurant on Friday night that has your favorite chocolate torte then be sure to stick to your nutrition plan on Monday, Tuesday, Wednesday, and Thursday, and enjoy your night out on Friday. Once Saturday morning arrives, do not have the "I ruined everything last night so who cares what I eat today" attitude. Another key concept of postpartum weight loss is getting right back on the wagon after taking a controlled step off it.

Principle (13) If You are Vegan or Vegetarian, Get Your Protein

As a vegan or vegetarian, look for high protein alternatives and eliminate items such as bread, pasta, crackers, and cereals. If your diet consists of a large majority of these gluten-containing foods, postpartum weight loss and maintenance may be difficult. High-carbohydrate foods such as bread, pasta, crackers, and cereal quickly convert into sugar which turns into fat if not used for energy. High protein vegan/vegetarian items can be found easily in most grocery stores. These products include quinoa, tempeh, beans, lentils, raw nuts, raw peanut butter, raw almond butter, split pea soup, vegetarian protein powder (blend with almond milk, banana, and strawberries for a delicious shake!), vegetarian chili, and hummus.

Principle (14) Avoid "Train Gain"

If you have been cleared to exercise by your doctor, avoid the big mistake of overeating—you will still gain weight, despite the fact you are working out. The average person's workout will only burn around 500 calories so it is imperative to stick to your nutrition regimen after an exercise session. Too many ice cream rewards for a job well done at the gym will backfire and negate all of the hard work you have put in.

We have all heard that people who work out need to "carb up" and eat more calories to have enough energy. This may be true for extremely competitive Ironman triathletes or Olympic athletes but if you're working out like a typical person (jogging eight miles per week or spending six hours per week in the gym), there is no physical need to store away excess carbohydrates to be used for energy. Keep in mind, to lose one pound of weight per week, you must cut out 500 calories from your daily intake. If you spend an hour exercising, you can reach this 500-calorie deficit and your work is done for the day. If you return home from the gym and reward yourself with four slices of pizza (1300 calories) instead of a sensible 600-calorie meal, you are now in excess of 800 calories.

Not working out? Replace a morning scone with oatmeal and an afternoon soda with iced tea and there's your 500-calorie deficit!

Principle ⑮ Eat Protein with Every Meal and Snack

Incorporating protein (animal and/or vegan) in every meal and snack will assist with weight management, muscle building, and toning (if you are one who is strength training). Proteins convert into amino acids and amino acids help to build muscle. Muscle assists with fat-burning and it's denser than fat so it takes up less space! In addition, protein consumption helps to keep your blood sugar levels even, which assists with preventing cravings. Some examples of my favorite proteins are eggs, broccoli, quinoa, nuts, beans, lentils, chicken, fish, shrimp, canned tuna, lean beef, turkey, and Greek yogurt.

Principle ⑯ Eat Good Fats

Most people do not consume enough omega-3 fatty acids because only a limited number of foods contain them. Omega-3 fats are not produced by our bodies so we need to get them from our diet—they assist with brain function, heart health, and reducing inflammation. Like protein, good fats also help our blood sugar levels to remain even and they can help us feel full for longer. Some examples of foods that have good fats are flaxseed, oysters, salmon, walnuts, mackerel, and avocado.

Principle ⑰ Keep it Simple

Nutrition can be complicated and overwhelming but if you implement these seven pillars into your daily routine, postpartum weight loss will happen for you!

- Control portions
- Focus on nutrient-dense foods

- Use green vegetables and low sugar fruits as a primary carbohydrate and fiber source
- Eliminate or severely limit gluten-containing carbohydrates
- Eliminate or limit added sugars

- Eat good fats
- Get your protein
- Exercise if your doctor has cleared you to do so
- Make a plan, prepare, and stick to the guidelines.

Postpartum Weight Loss Guidelines

Green Vegetables (at least four servings per day): some examples are broccoli, asparagus, kale, spinach, collard greens, celery, artichoke, and Brussels sprouts.

Proteins (at least three servings per day): some examples are chicken, fish, canned tuna, turkey, Greek yogurt, beef, tempeh, natto, nuts, beans, lentils, broccoli, and quinoa.

Low-Sugar Fruits (two to three servings per day): some examples are blueberries, raspberries, blackberries, tomato, apricot, grapefruit, and avocado.

Healthy Fats (two to three servings per day): some examples are avocado, walnuts, chia seeds, extra-virgin olive oil, wild salmon, and grass-fed beef.

Probiotic Foods* (zero to one serving per day): some examples are Greek yogurt, kefir, coconut kefir, brine-cured olives, sauerkraut, kimchi, natto, tempeh, and apple cider vinegar.

*See Chapter 4 for probiotic supplement information to substitute for these foods.

Starchy Produce (zero to one serving per day): some examples are sweet potato, butternut squash, fingerling potatoes, parsnips, and pumpkin.

Everyone is different, so you may drop your baby weight in a few weeks, a few months, or maybe not for a year—just stick to the plan, be consistent, and be patient! Keep in mind, if you are nursing, you will need a few hundred (give or take) extra calories per day as opposed to someone who is not nursing. In the following chapter, we will provide nursing mothers with tips to help increase milk supply while safely losing the baby weight.

Chapter 14
Dietary Recommendations for Nursing

Those who are nursing may be wondering if you can lose the baby weight while still maintaining your milk supply. Everyone is different but yes, it is most definitely possible if you eat enough (but not too many) calories from nutrient-dense foods. There are many theories about how to maintain a milk supply; I will go over these alternatives and I'll tell you the ones I employed that may have worked for me. I exclusively breast-fed my son until he was eight months old and continued until he was a toddler, all while maintaining my milk supply as well as my pre-pregnancy weight. The strategies I used to build and uphold my milk supply may have been beneficial, but a lot of evidence regarding these tactics are anecdotal without any conclusive research. The one strategy that I positively swear by for exceptional milk production is proper nutrition; however, I will go over additional options as well since they may help you!

Since you are nursing, you are probably getting a lot of conflicting nutrition advice just like you did during pregnancy. The good news is that nutrition for nursing is not that complicated—you don't need to spend lots of time seeking out special groceries or preparing certain meals. Of course, I recommend balanced nutrition like the information you have found in this book; however, your diet does not have to be perfect to provide and maintain nutritious breast milk. Regardless of the mother's diet, many components of the breast milk will stay consistent as whatever you are lacking in your diet, tends to be made up for via the stores in your body. I still recommend eating nutrient-dense foods as you will need your energy while taking care of your new baby and you do not want all of your own nutrition stores stripped from your body, so it is best to replenish it with beneficial macro- and micro-nutrients. If you are a vegan or vegetarian, it is imperative to speak to your doctor or lactation consultant about possibly supplementing vitamin B12 since that is found in animal products and the levels found in your breast milk can be altered by your diet.

I'm not a certified lactation consultant but I will pass on the most important piece of advice from my own lactation consultant, which helped me greatly. To produce milk, nurse your baby (or pump) frequently. Your baby's sucking and the emptying of your breasts will prompt them to refill.

In addition to eating nutrient-dense foods, I recommend staying hydrated, with water as your primary beverage. Being mindful of your body's thirst and drinking fluids when you feel thirsty is a must. Despite some mainstream statements, there is no conclusive evidence that shows drinking excess fluids (beyond what your body needs) will increase your milk production. I highly recommend against one of the most common suggestions that nursing mothers receive, and that faulty advice is to drink sports drinks for hydration and electrolyte replenishment. Popular sports drinks contain a variety of sweeteners such as high-fructose corn syrup and liquefied table sugar which will not assist your postpartum weight loss

efforts. Even more alarming, some sports drinks contain harmful chemicals such as brominated vegetable oil. Brominated vegetable oil is a combination of bromine and vegetable oil and is similar in composition to brominated flame retardants; this additive is used to remove any cloudiness to the appearance of the beverage. Banned in Japan and Europe, consumption of brominated vegetable oil is associated with thyroid disease, memory loss, fatigue, tremors, skin rashes, cancer, and hormone disorders.

Sports drinks are suggested to nursing mothers for electrolyte replacement—but the risks outweigh the benefits. Electrolytes are minerals such as calcium, potassium, sodium, and magnesium, and we do excrete this through our breastmilk, sweat, and urine, so yes, it is important to replenish these minerals. You can do so by eating mineral-containing foods including but not limited to vegetables, fruits, beans, fish, and meats. To get hydration and electrolytes all in one, try some of these delicious combinations.

① **Chia Seeds and Raw Coconut Water**
Raw coconut water is relatively low in sugar and boasts a variety of electrolytes. Stirring

in a tablespoon of chia seeds will add some texture as well as protein, omega-3 fatty acids, and fiber.

(2) **Almond Milk, Spinach, and Banana**
This combination provides calcium, magnesium, potassium, as well as folate, Vitamin A, and iron! Simply blend one cup almond milk, one frozen banana, and one cup raw spinach. Feel free to add a pinch of sea salt for sodium, though most of us obtain enough salt in our diets and adding more probably isn't necessary.

(3) **Celery, Ginger, Lemon, and Apple**
If you have a juicer or go to juice bars where you can choose your own ingredients, juice five stalks of celery, a few pieces of ginger, one lemon, and half an apple. This drink is light and refreshing with a limited amount of sugar and contains naturally occurring sodium, phosphorus, chloride, magnesium, and potassium.

During your nursing journey, you may feel like your supply is waning, but it may be perfectly fine as our bodies tend to regulate based on the baby's needs. If you truly feel something is off and you're not able to feed your baby enough, it is best to see your doctor and lactation consultant in case there are any underlying causes that may be negatively affecting your milk production. If you have checked out fine but you just want to experiment with boosting your supply, the following recommendations don't have solid conclusive evidence that shows a correlation between consumption and supply increase, however, many lactating women do swear by these tactics. I will present some commonly used alternatives and you can decide if you would like to try any of them!

First of all, prolactin is a hormone which helps to produce breast milk. There are foods and herbs that are considered galactagogues which increase prolactin levels, resulting in supposed stimulation of milk production. Some widely used galactagogue foods include:

- Oatmeal
- Garlic
- Fennel
- Dark, leafy greens such as kale, spinach, collard greens, and broccoli
- Garbanzo beans
- Ginger
- Almonds
- Papaya

- Some spices such as turmeric and fennel seeds
- Gluten-free brewer's yeast

If you are not familiar with brewer's yeast, it is made with a one-celled fungus and is commonly known as a galactagogue in the breastfeeding community. Traditional brewer's yeast is found in beer and is not considered gluten-free, however there are gluten-free versions on the market that are made from non-GMO sugar beet molasses. Easily utilized in shakes and recipes, gluten-free brewer's yeast offers one of the richest sources of vitamins and trace elements.

The above mentioned are *Whole Food Pregnancy*–approved, so feel free to add these into your diet (if you haven't done so already) for possible milk production increase. I personally ate an abundance of most of these foods during my breastfeeding journey and although I have no proof that it resulted in over two years of successful breastfeeding, I do feel that it helped, not only my milk but my overall energy levels and postpartum weight loss. For your convenience, *The Whole Food Pregnancy Plan* recipes found in Chapters 17, 18, 19, and 20 incorporate many of these ingredients in several recipes.

More controversial galactagogues are herbs. With regard to lactation, most herbal treatments have not been comprehensively researched. I am presenting this information in a non-biased manner and urge you to do your own research and consult with your doctor or lactation consultant before starting an herbal treatment regimen. The following herbs are some of the most popular, widely consumed by lactating mothers but once again, the efficacy of herbal treatments is more anecdotal as opposed to research-based.

④ Red Raspberry Leaf Tea

Red Raspberry Leaf tea is an herbal tea that is naturally caffeine-free and can be found in most major grocery stores. According to the American Pregnancy Association, this tea promotes uterine health when consumed during pregnancy (avoid during the first trimester) and helps increase milk production when nursing. Studies have shown this iron-rich tea is safe to consume while nursing as well as during the second and third trimesters of pregnancy.

⑤ Fenugreek

Fenugreek is commonly consumed by nursing mothers to increase milk supply and has been around for centuries. Many nursing women have reported seeing an increase in their milk supplies within three days of starting this herbal treatment and many have reported seeing no change in their milk supplies. Fenugreek is a common food ingredient found in curries and chutneys and is on the US Food and Drug Administration's safe list when consumed in moderation.

⑥ Blessed Thistle

Originally from the Mediterranean, blessed thistle has been used in herbal medicine since the Middle Ages. Blessed thistle can be found in breastfeeding teas or in capsule form. According to the American Pregnancy Association, blessed thistle is most effective when taken in combination with fenugreek. Many commercially-prepared lactation teas which are catered to nursing women include both blessed thistle and fenugreek.

There have been reports from numerous breastfeeding women that the above-mentioned herbs increased their milk supplies after as little as three days of use. The above herbs can be found at your local health foods store or online. If you choose to try herbs to increase your milk supply (after consulting with your health care provider or lactation consultant), be sure to follow recommended doses that are provided on the labels.

If you haven't heard of lactation cookies yet, I'm sure you will in the near future! Lactation cookies are extremely popular in the nursing community, though I advise against *most* of them. The majority of lactation cookies host a variety of ingredients that are not beneficial for postpartum weight loss (such as sugar and flour) and only offer one or two ingredients that may be beneficial to your milk supply. So you can spot lactation cookies that may *sabotage* your postpartum weight loss goals, below is a popular lactation cookie ingredients list that I advise *against*.

1 cup butter
1 cup sugar
1 cup firmly packed brown sugar
4 tablespoons water
2 tablespoons flax seed meal
2 eggs
1 teaspoon vanilla
3 cups flour
1 teaspoon baking soda
1 teaspoon salt
3 cups oats
1 cup chocolate chips
2–4 tablespoons brewer's yeast

The ingredients that may be beneficial to your milk supply are the oats, flax seed meal, and brewer's yeast, but that only accounts for a small portion of this list! Having a batch of cookies around the house that contain this much sugar and flour will not make postpartum weight loss an easy task. You can easily use oats, flax seed, and gluten-free brewer's yeast in a nutritious shake by combining the following ingredients in a blender.

1 frozen banana
¼ cup dry oats
½ cup almond milk or coconut water
1 tablespoon flaxseed meal
1 tablespoon gluten-free brewer's yeast
1 dollop real peanut or almond butter

If lactation cookies sound like a fun idea to you and you love to bake, this recipe is *Whole Food Pregnancy*–approved and the cookies are delicious! The following recipe will yield around thirty mid-sized cookies and they will each be around 120 calories. Enjoy!

Ingredients:

3 large, ripe bananas (mashed)
5 tablespoons honey or agave
1 teaspoon vanilla extract
6 tablespoons real almond or peanut butter
½ cup coconut oil
3 tablespoons cocoa nibs
20 pecans or almonds, finely chopped
3 cups raw oats
3 tablespoons ground flax seed
⅔ cup almond flour
2 tablespoons gluten-free brewer's yeast
1 teaspoon cinnamon
1 teaspoon baking powder

Directions:

1. Pre-heat oven to 350° F.

2. Thoroughly combine the mashed banana with honey or agave, vanilla, peanut or almond butter, and coconut oil (warm the coconut oil to get it into a liquid state before combining with other ingredients).

3. In a different bowl, combine all of the dry ingredients and then mix the dry ingredients with the wet ingredients.

4. Using your hands, make balls of dough and place them on a parchment-lined baking sheet. Gently press the balls down to flatten.

5. Bake on one side for 9 minutes and then turn them over; continue baking for 7 more minutes.

6. The cookies will harden as they cool.

7. If you prefer uncooked cookie bites, you can skip the baking step. Simply roll the raw dough into balls and proceed to roll them in shredded coconut. Keep frozen or refrigerated until you are ready to eat them.

Some women choose to incorporate all of the tactics exhibited in this chapter while others only try one or even none. Overall, one of the most beneficial approaches you can take while nursing is to maintain proper nutrition as you will be healthier with ample amounts of energy which is important for your own well-being while raising your newborn. Listening to your body, eating when you are hungry, drinking to meet your thirst, and nursing/pumping very frequently is key. If you need assistance, most hospitals provide lactation consultants who can advise you during your breastfeeding journey. Good luck!

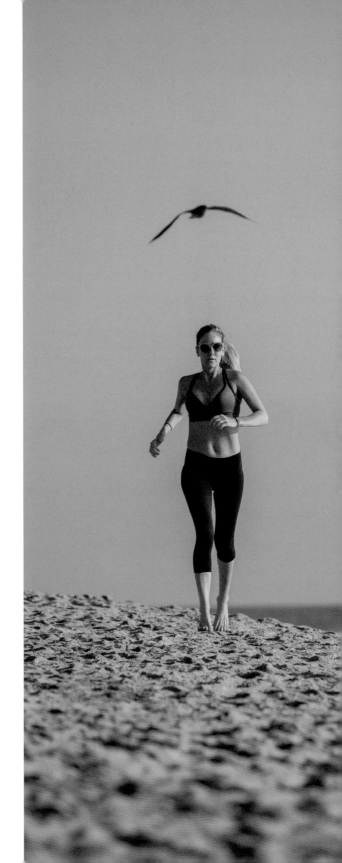

Chapter 15
What Not to Feed Your Infant

When my son was as young as ten months old, we would get looks of astonishment from other restaurant patrons when they noticed him eating exactly what my husband and I were eating—foods such as fish, Brussels sprouts, and tomato. Many people believe that babies and young children will only eat bland items such as crackers and cereal or sweet items such as fruit purees and squeezable yogurts. This may be true for many little ones if they have been conditioned from a very young age to eat processed, high-carbohydrate, and high-sugar foods that have been labeled as "baby food." This conditioning of taste buds is likely to result in aversions to green vegetables and other nutrient-dense items, leading to potentially negative life-long nutrition habits. You can train your baby's taste buds to enjoy fare such as broccoli, fish, avocado, tomatoes, and lentils. The first step is to avoid baby cereals.

Back in the 1950s, baby food companies launched a genius advertising campaign which boasted the nutrition benefits of infant cereals. Due to the highly successful marketing strategies of these companies (which were driven solely for the purpose of raising their own profit margins), this "wisdom" has been passed along by nutritionists and doctors for more than sixty years. In fact, there is no scientific evidence which shows that baby cereal is

> These grain-based cereals are full of ingredients that a baby's immature GI system is unable to process. If you picture a baby's gut as a long tunnel, imagine that it is full of holes. Breastmilk closes these holes, reducing the risk of foodborne allergies and sensitivities. Formula does not have the same ability to close these gaps, making it even more important for formula-fed babies to avoid solids before they are ready.
>
> **—Katie Williams, RN**

beneficial to the growth and development of infants. A few facts about baby cereals:

- They are highly processed and have incredibly long shelf lives.
- The majority of the nutrients are fortified, meaning they are fake and do not absorb as well as naturally occurring nutrients you will find in whole foods.
- They are grain-based and babies under the age of one cannot digest grains efficiently due to their lack of the enzyme amylase, which breaks down starches.
- The main ingredients are different types of flours and rice; flour and rice are high glycemic, meaning they will convert to sugar (and lots of it) soon after consumption.
- The type of carbohydrates found in baby cereals have been associated with the increased development of type II diabetes, insulin resistance, and heart disease in adults.
- Early consumption of these highly processed, high-glycemic carbohydrates found in baby cereals may prime a little one's palate to lead to the dependence on processed, high-carb foods such as breads, pastas, cookies, and pastries throughout childhood and adulthood.

One question I am asked repeatedly is, "When should I introduce gluten into my baby's diet?" My answer is, never, especially if that child is a gene carrier. Preventing a disease by avoiding the grains that cause celiac disease is just good and easy advice. Treating food as medicine, or potential poison, is not a new concept, but it is certainly one that has been neglected in our world until most recently. Everyone has to eat and what you choose to eat can have the most profound effect on your health and the health of your children. Repeated research articles have proven that it doesn't matter when, how much, or at what age you expose your infant to gluten in the expression of celiac disease and NCGS.

—Nadine Grzeskowiak, RN, BSN, CEN

In addition to baby cereals, jarred baby foods run rampant on the shelves of United States grocery stores. In fact, American babies consume an average of 600 jars of baby food before the age of one, which is three times the amount of baby food compared to European babies. Some baby food manufacturers do use suitable ingredients which can be acceptable choices for your baby, however we advise against making jarred baby food a staple that is regularly implemented in your baby's diet. These types of foods are highly processed so they tend to have tastes and textures that are unlike the natural source of the particular food. When a baby is only accustomed to purees, he/she may find it difficult to enjoy and transition to unprocessed versions of proteins and vegetables. On one occasion, I purchased a jar of organic baby food (pureed peas) and my son, who was ten months old at the time, refused to eat it despite the fact he had been eating a variety of vegetables and legumes for two months prior. I was curious so I tried the baby food myself, and the taste and texture was nothing like what he was used to (or what I was used to), so I understood the reason for his aversion. Now, if you take that scenario and flip-flop it (only feed your baby highly-processed purees), it may be likely that he/she will be opposed to real food in its natural form as it will be very foreign.

If you are going to use jarred baby food (yes, they are very convenient and time can be scarce when you're a parent!), I highly recommend reading the ingredient labels, as many of the food titles do not accurately reflect what you will find in the jar. Even organic brands may use fillers such as water and wheat-based flours so

the manufacturer can make more food with less expensive ingredients. Not only does this tactic dilute the nutritional properties of the food, it also results in the consumption of wheat- and rice-based flours. Before the age of one (and sometimes not until the age of two), infants do not produce enough amylase (an enzyme that breaks down carbohydrates) to digest certain starches and grains. When an infant cannot properly digest a given food, he/she will not acquire nutritional benefits from it and may develop an upset stomach. Below you will find three examples of popular, relied-upon organic jarred baby food that is intended for infant consumption. Despite the fact they are marketed as meals containing only protein, vegetables, and sweet potato, you will find grain-based fillers in all three.

Harvest Squash Turkey from Leading Organic Brand: Organic Butternut Squash, Water, Organic Ground Turkey, Organic Whole Grain Kamut Flour (Wheat), Organic Whole Grain Quinoa Flour. CONTAINS WHEAT.

Zucchini Broccoli Medley from Leading Organic Brand: Organic Vegetables (Organic Zucchini, Organic Peas, Organic

Broccoli), Water, Organic Whole Wheat Couscous. CONTAINS: WHEAT.

Sweet Potato and Chicken from Leading Organic Brand:
Organic Sweet Potatoes, Water, Organic Whole Grain Brown Rice Flour, Organic Apricot Puree, Organic Ground Chicken.

Other processed items including but not limited to teething biscuits, puffs, and squeezable tubes of yogurt have become mainstream and acceptable sources of nutrition for babies. These foods are touted as having the nutrients your baby needs as well as being convenient for the parents. Let's take a look at the ingredients in the above-mentioned foods that have become commonplace in the diets of millions of babies and toddlers.

Teething Biscuits from a Leading Brand of Baby Foods:
Whole Wheat Flour, Enriched Flour (Wheat Flour, Niacin, Iron, Thiamin Mononitrate, Riboflavin, Folic Acid), Sugar, Ultra-Low Linolenic Soybean Oil And/Or High Oleic Canola Oil and/or High Oleic Sunflower Oil, Whey (From Milk), Calcium Carbonate, Molasses, Salt, Ammonium Bicarbonate, Vanilla Extract, Sodium Bicarbonate, Alpha Tocopherol Acetate (Vitamin E), Ferric

Orthophosphate (Iron), Mixed Tocopherols (For Freshness), Zinc Oxide, Natural Butter Flavor, Electrolytic Iron, Soy Lecithin.

Squeezable Strawberry Yogurt from a Leading Yogurt Brand:
Cultured Pasteurized Grade a Low Fat Milk, Sugar, Modified Corn Starch, Kosher Gelatin, Tricalcium Phosphate, Potassium Sorbate, Carrageenan, Natural and Artificial Flavor, Vegetable and Fruit Juice (For Color), Vitamin A Acetate, Vitamin D3.

Strawberry Apple Puffs from a Leading Brand of Baby Foods:
Rice Flour, whole wheat flour, wheat starch, cane sugar, whole grain oat flour, dried apple puree, less than 2 percent of: natural strawberry apple flavor (includes strawberry and apple juice concentrates), calcium phosphate, mixed tocopherols (to maintain freshness), sunflower lecithin.

Based on the ingredients lists of the above items, you can see they are highly processed with many additives and preservatives. Let's take a further look at a few of the ingredients that I, as a nutritionist, find particularly alarming not only for baby consumption but for human consumption in general. Please read the ingredient labels of foods you may be intending to purchase for your baby as it may be best to steer clear of items that contain the following.

Soybean Oil: Since 94 percent of all soybeans grown in the United States are genetically modified, it is highly likely that soybean oil found in packaged items is coming from genetically modified soybeans. If you're not familiar with the term GMO (genetically modified organism), to put it simply, this means that these soybeans have been altered so they can withstand being sprayed with lethal doses of the herbicide Roundup, which contains glyphosate. When we consume these soybeans or the oil from them, we are also consuming glyphosate, which according to some studies is linked to conditions such as cancer, multiple sclerosis, infertility, allergies, and cardiovascular disease (read more about GMOs on page 92).

Soy Lecithin: This is an additive in many processed foods that serves as an emulsifier, making the appearance of the foods more visually appealing in terms of being smooth and uniform. The chemical solvent hexane is used to extract the oil from the soybeans; traces of the neurotoxin hexane are found in products containing soy lecithin. Many studies have cited diarrhea, stomach pain, bloating, and rashes as side effects of soy lecithin consumption.

Sugar: Too much sugar is the primary cause for obesity and type II Diabetes so it is imperative to avoid baby and toddler foods with added sugars. The foods you introduce to your little one will establish a pattern of eating that may continue on through adulthood so avoiding added sugars is imperative. Also look for sugar in disguise; it may be listed as Anhydrous dextrose, brown rice syrup, cane crystals, corn syrup, crystal dextrose, evaporated cane juice, fruit juice concentrate, high-fructose corn syrup, honey, liquid fructose, malt syrup, maple syrup, or molasses.

Carrageenan: This is a food additive that is used as an emulsifier to improve the texture of many processed foods. The trade lobby group for carrageenan fought for it to remain in organic foods as well so you will see it in items such as organic infant formulas. Several studies have linked the consumption of carrageenan to diabetes, cancer, and inflammation.

To avoid these above-mentioned ingredients that are found in an abundance of popular baby foods, I suggest the following guidelines:

- Choose whole foods that occur in nature.
- Choose foods that have naturally occurring vitamins and minerals as opposed to fortified synthetic vitamins.
- Avoid foods that are packaged and have long shelf lives.
- Avoid foods with added sugars.
- Avoid foods that have ingredient labels with more than four ingredients.
- Avoid foods that have ingredients you cannot pronounce.
- Be open to preparing your own baby foods and snacks.

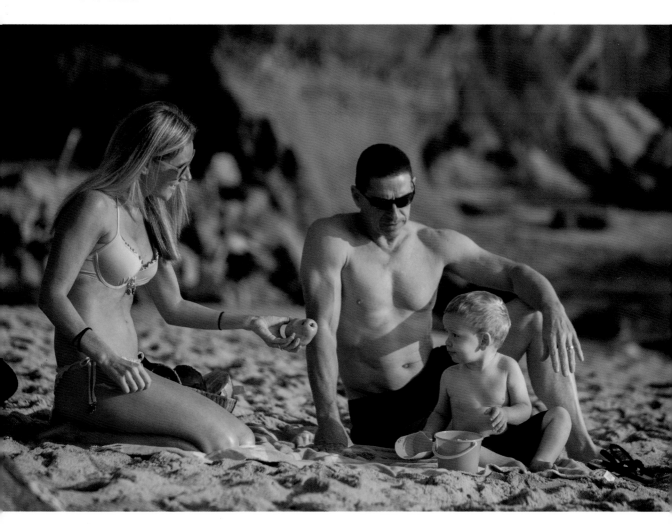

Chapter 16
Baby's First Solids

So what, exactly, should baby's first solids be? First of all, I don't recommend introducing solids until six months of age, and keep in mind that some babies may not be ready for solids until a little later than that. First solids should be given in conjunction with breast milk and/or formula as infants under the age of one still need the added nutrition from those sources.

Many pediatricians recommend "solids" (i.e., purees and baby cereals) far too early, often at only four months of age, sometimes even as early as six weeks. The results of this can be extremely detrimental to a baby's health, leading to a lifetime of allergies and food sensitivities (ever wonder why you can't tolerate gluten?).[72] Most babies will indicate a desire to start solids sometime between six and eight months of age. It's important to keep in mind that "Food before one is just for fun," and that infants under one year of age still need to be getting the bulk of their calories and nutrients from breast milk or formula.[73] A primary reason many parents ignore the current advice to wait until six months is the desire for the infant to sleep longer at night. Studies have shown that feeding young babies solids before bed does *not* lead to better sleep. In fact, it may have the opposite effect by causing stomach upset and gas as the infant's immature GI system struggles to digest foreign ingredients. In one large study, babies fed more calories during the day *did* feed less at night, but had the same amount of night awakenings as those not yet on solids.[74]

—Katie Williams, RN

72 J. Scott et al., "Predictors of the early introduction of solid foods in infants: results of a cohort study," NCBI, September 22, 2009, accessed September 29, 2017, https://www.ncbi.nlm.nih.gov/pmc/articles/PMC2754451/.
73 J. Scott et al., "Predictors of the early introduction of solid foods in infants: results of a cohort study," NCBI, September 22, 2009, accessed September 29, 2017, https://www.ncbi.nlm.nih.gov/pmc/articles/PMC2754451/.
74 A. Brown and V. Harries, "Infant Sleep and Night Feeding Patterns During Later Infancy: Association with Breastfeeding Frequency, Daytime Complementary Food Intake, and Infant Weight," Mary Anne Liebert, Inc. Publishers, June 09, 2015, , accessed September 29, 2017, http://online.liebertpub.com/doi/10.1089/bfm.2014.0153.

Baby-Led Weaning is the process of adding complementary foods to a baby's breast milk or formula diet. It bypasses the typical stage of pureed foods and instead allows baby to eat the same foods her parents are eating, just in finger-food size. "But what about choking!?!" you might exclaim. When babies naturally start reaching for foods on their parents' plates, this is an indicator that they are physically and developmentally ready to eat solids. A baby should be able to sit up on her own, hold her head up with good neck control, and should be babbling. These are signs that the baby has the muscular development necessary to manipulate food in her mouth, and is a sign that internally, her gastrointestinal system is mature enough to accept food other than milk. In addition, a baby may "gag" on a food without actually choking on it. The gag reflex is a warning that food is getting too close to the trachea (breathing pipe) and helps the baby manipulate the food into a better chewing position. This gag reflex actually starts out closer to the front of the mouth in infants under one year, gradually moving back as they age. This further prevents actual choking episodes (which are rarely reported by parents who have used BLW).[75]

—**Katie Williams, RN**

For one of your baby's very first solid foods, I recommend cooked egg yolk. (Please note to omit the egg white as the white of an egg may cause an allergic reaction in babies who are younger than one year of age.) If your baby doesn't like the chalky texture of a cooked egg yolk, try mashing it with a sprinkle of water until the consistency is smooth. If your baby still isn't a fan, mash one half of a very ripe banana and thoroughly combine with one egg yolk until you have a batter-like consistency and scramble your banana-egg yolk mixture over medium heat—this will be sure to delight your little one! Egg yolks boast the following:

- Long-chain fatty acids which are imperative to the development of the baby's nervous system and brain.
- Protein! It is a misconception that all of the protein is in the egg white; the yolk contains HALF of the egg's total protein.
- Egg yolks contain the enzyme amylase which is needed to break down starches.

75 G. Rapley and T. Murkett, *Baby-Led Weaning: The Essential Guide to Introducing Solid Foods* (New York, NY: Workman Publishing, 2010).

Other first solids I recommend are categorized by age below:

Six months of age

FOOD	BENEFITS
Egg Yolk	Easily digested; contains good fats and fat soluble vitamins A, D, E, K; contains choline, vitamin B12, thiamin, riboflavin, folate, zinc, copper, and selenium; contain protein.
Sweet Potato	Easily digested and aid in digestion of other foods; contains beta carotene, iron and phosphorus; contains vitamins B1, B2, B6, and C; contains antioxidants to fight inflammation.
Organic Berries (blueberries, blackberries, raspberries, strawberries)	Contains vitamin C, folate, magnesium, vitamin B, riboflavin, thiamine, riboflavin, dietary fiber, and antioxidants.
Avocado	High in good fats; contains folate, calcium, magnesium, phosphorus, and vitamin C.
Banana	Contains potassium, vitamin A, vitamin B6, vitamin C, calcium, magnesium, iron, and zinc; contains pectin to aid with digestion.
Cooked Butternut Squash	Easily digested, contains vitamins A and C, vitamin B6, calcium, magnesium, and fiber.
Cooked Green Peas	Contains vitamins A, C, and K, manganese, folate, fiber, vitamin B1, copper, phosphorus, iron, protein, and choline.

Low iron (anemia) can cause Restless Leg Syndrome in both children and adults. This can lead to sleep disturbances as children become so restless that they wake themselves up. Other signs of anemia are increased illness (due to lower immune system), fatigue, and pale skin. Dietary iron is absorbed at a much higher rate than the iron found in vitamins, and has the added advantage of not causing nearly as much constipation and stomach upset as iron supplements.[76]

—Katie Williams, RN

76   C. Dosman, M. Witmans, and L. Zwaigenbaum, "Iron's role in paediatric restless legs syndrome-a review," NCBI, April 2012, , accessed September 29, 2017, https://www.ncbi.nlm.nih.gov/pmc/articles/PMC3381661/.

Eight months of age

FOOD	BENEFITS
All foods found in the six-month category	See above.
Cooked Green Vegetables (broccoli, asparagus, Brussels sprouts, kale, collard greens, spinach)	Vitamins A, C, E, and K, chromium, folate, fiber, pantothenic acid, vitamin B6, vitamin E, manganese, selenium, choline, pantothenic acid, niacin, potassium, phosphorus, choline, vitamins B1 and B2, copper, omega-3 fatty acids, protein, calcium, and iron.
Cooked Carrots	Vitamins A, C, E, and K, biotin, fiber, molybdenum, potassium, vitamins B1 and B2, manganese, niacin, pantothenic acid, phosphorus, folate, and copper.
Cooked Cauliflower	Vitamins C and K, protein, niacin, thiamin, riboflavin, magnesium, phosphorus, fiber, vitamin B6, potassium, folate, and pantothenic acid.
Low-Sugar Fruits (apple, apricot, tomato, bell pepper)	Vitamins A, C, E, and K, pectin, fiber, biotin, molybdenum, copper, potassium, manganese, fiber, vitamins B2 and B6, folate, niacin, phosphorus, and, carotenoids.
Hummus	Vitamins C, E, and K; vitamin B6; protein; manganese, copper, calcium, iron, magnesium, zinc, folate, and thiamin.
Cooked Lentils	Vitamins B1 and B6, potassium, zinc, pantothenic acid, molybdenum, folate, fiber, copper, phosphorus, manganese, iron, and protein.
Beans (black, pinto, lima, kidney)	Vitamins A, C, and K, protein, thiamin, riboflavin, niacin, Vitamin B6, calcium, iron, magnesium, phosphorus, potassium, copper, manganese, folate, and fiber.
Mushrooms	Vitamins C and D, thiamin, magnesium, Vitamin B6, folate, fiber, riboflavin, niacin, pantothenic acid, iron, phosphorus, potassium, zinc, copper, manganese, and selenium.
Organic Grass-fed Beef	Vitamins B3, B6, and B12; protein, omega-3 fatty acids, selenium, iron, zinc, phosphorus, choline, and pantothenic acid.
Turkey Breast	Vitamins B2, B3, B6, and B12; protein, iron, selenium, zinc, phosphorus, choline, and pantothenic acid.
Wild Salmon	Vitamin D; vitamins B6 and B12; selenium, niacin, phosphorus, choline, biotin, pantothenic acid, and potassium; protein and omega-3 fatty acids.
Wild White Fish (Halibut, Sole, Rockfish, Mahi Mahi, Opah)	Vitamin D, vitamins B5, B6, and B12, magnesium, potassium, niacin, phosphorus, and selenium; protein.
Chicken	Vitamins B6 and B12; niacin, selenium, phosphorus, choline, and pantothenic acid; protein.

*At 12 months of age, consult with your pediatrician about adding additional foods into your baby's diet such as the whole egg (egg white included), nut butters, shell fish, and other possible food allergens.

Babies and toddlers between the ages of nine and eighteen months are at the greatest risk for iron-deficiency—a common cause for this is diet. Babies are usually born with enough stores of iron to get them through the first six months of life but after that, they may need a little iron boost. My son was almost exclusively breast fed (with the exception of trying a few solids for fun) until the age of nine months. Although the iron found in breast milk is easily absorbed, there still isn't a lot of it! At my son's nine-month well visit, his iron levels came in at the low end of normal and we were advised to administer iron supplements as any further drop in the iron level would possibly be cause for concern. We decided to forgo the supplements, concentrating on iron-rich foods from animal- and plant-based sources, and we were pleased to find that his iron levels had skyrocketed by the next well visit! Below are the iron-rich foods we implemented on a regular basis for our nine-month-old (and still do to this day at the age of three years). The Institute of Medicine recommends 11 milligrams of iron per day for infants ages six to twelvemonths. Also, for the most efficient iron absorption, pair these foods with sources of vitamin C such as berries, tomato, bell pepper, broccoli, and citrus fruits.

FOOD	IRON (mg)
Chicken Liver (2 Ounces)	7
Beef Liver (2 Ounces)	3
Venison (2 Ounces)	2.5
Beef (2 Ounces)	1.7
Cooked Spinach (¼ Cup)	1.6
Cooked Lentils (¼ Cup)	1.6
Hummus (¼ Cup)	1.4
Cooked Lima Beans (¼ Cup)	1.1
Cooked Black-Eyed Peas (¼ Cup)	1.1
Cooked Pinto Beans (¼ Cup)	0.8
Wild Salmon (2 Ounces)	0.7
Chicken (2 Ounces)	0.7
Turkey Breast (2 Ounces)	0.6
Cooked Green Peas (¼Cup)	0.6
Egg Yolk (1 Yolk)	0.5

Of course, many infants/toddlers won't have the ability or desire to eat something like cooked spinach. A trick I used was to blend roasted sweet potato, cooked spinach, and cooked turkey breast with a little bit of extra-virgin olive oil in a food processor; the texture is baby-friendly and many will love the taste of the sweet potato.

*Disclaimer—some levels of iron deficiency may require medical attention; consult your doctor.

- Breast milk provides natural antibodies that help your baby avoid illnesses such as acute and prolonged diarrhea, respiratory tract infections, otitis media, urinary tract infection, neonatal septicemia, and necrotizing enterocolitis. Studies suggest that this protection may last longer than the actual act of breastfeeding.[77]
- Breastfed babies are often less constipated and gassy due to the enzymes found in breast milk that aid in digestion.[78]
- Studies have shown that the risk of Sudden Infant Death Syndrome (SIDS) is greatly reduced in breast fed infants.[79]
- Breastfeeding for at least nine months has shown in some studies to significantly raise your child's cognition; this may be contributed to the fact that breast milk provides specific nutrients for the immature brain.[80]
- Breastfed babies are less likely to develop obesity, type 1 and type 2 diabetes, and leukemia later in life; nursing mothers are at lower risk for premenopausal breast cancer, ovarian cancer, retained gestational weight gain, type 2 diabetes, myocardial infarction, and the metabolic syndrome.[81]
- According to recent studies, active bonding during breastfeeding led to six-year-old children who displayed the lowest risks of internalizing behavior disorders such as anxiety and depression.[82]
- Breast milk is void of ingredients that commercial baby formula contains such as corn syrup, cow's milk, soy bean oil, vegetable oil, carrageenan, soy lecithin, and synthetic nutrients.

Breast milk is more than 80 percent water, so additional water is not necessary for the breastfeeding infant. The World Health Organization (WHO) recommends no water before the age of six months as this can lead to diarrhea, stomach upset, and malnutrition (as the water falsely fills baby up and replaces calories and nutrients from breast milk).[83]

—Katie Williams, RN

77 LA Hanson, "Breastfeeding provides passive and likely long-lasting active immunity.," NCBI, December 1998, accessed October 01, 2017, https://www.ncbi.nlm.nih.gov/pubmed/9892025.

78 LA Heitlinger, "Enzymes in mother's milk and their possible role in digestion.," NCBI, 1983, accessed October 01, 2017, https://www.ncbi.nlm.nih.gov/pubmed/6196470.

79 MM Vennemann et al., "Does breastfeeding reduce the risk of sudden infant death syndrome?" NCBI, March 2009, accessed October 01, 2017, https://www.ncbi.nlm.nih.gov/pubmed/19254976.

80 H. Lee et al., "Effect of Breastfeeding Duration on Cognitive Development in Infants: 3-Year Follow-up Study," NCBI, April 2016, accessed October 01, 2017, https://www.ncbi.nlm.nih.gov/pmc/articles/PMC4810341/.

81 A. Stuebe, "The Risks of Not Breastfeeding for Mothers and Infants," NCBI, 2009, accessed October 01, 2017, https://www.ncbi.nlm.nih.gov/pmc/articles/PMC2812877/.

82 J. Liu, P. Leung, and A. Yang, "Breastfeeding and Active Bonding Protects against Children's Internalizing Behavior Problems," NCBI, January 2014, accessed October 01, 2017, https://www.ncbi.nlm.nih.gov/pmc/articles/PMC3916850/.

83 "Why can't we give water to a breastfeeding baby before the 6 months, even when it is hot?" World Health Organization. July 2014. Accessed September 29, 2017. http://www.who.int/features/qa/breastfeeding/en/.

Beverages for Your Little One

Water is not recommended for babies under six months of age as they should be hydrating with breast milk or formula. As your baby reaches eight to ten months old, she may drink minimal amounts of water; however, breast milk and/or formula should still be the primary beverage. After the age of one year, water can be used if paired with nutrient-dense foods found in this chapter, but if possible, the incorporation of breast milk is still the most superior way to hydrate your twelve-month old.

According to The American Academy of Pediatrics (AAP), breast milk is the best nutrition for infants, so babies should be fed breast milk exclusively for the first six months of life. Even after solids have been introduced, the AAP promotes breast milk consumption until at least one year of age, and even longer, given that both baby and mother find it mutually beneficial. The following are substantial benefits of infant/toddler breast milk consumption:

Many doctors advise to start integrating a consistent amount of cow's milk into a one-year-old's diet. Like the marketing of baby cereals, the marketing of cow's milk has been quite extensive, leading the masses to believe that it is a superior beverage due to its calcium, added vitamin D, and protein. To the contrary, studies are now suggesting that cow's milk should be avoided or limited due to the following:

- According to the US National Library of Medicine, the casein and calcium present in cow's milk inhibits iron absorption.[84]
- An overabundance of calories from cow's milk may lead to less consumption of other nutrient-dense foods.
- Infant consumption of cow's milk puts her at higher risk for dehydration, resulting from excessive protein and minerals found in cow's milk needing to be excreted through urine.[85]
- Modern cows lactate while they are pregnant, which results in elevated estrogen levels in milk which has been linked with early sexual maturation in children, lower testosterone

---

84 EE Ziegler, "Consumption of cow's milk as a cause of iron deficiency in infants and toddlers." NCBI, November 2011, accessed September 10, 2017, https://www.ncbi.nlm.nih.gov/pubmed/22043881.\

85 EE Ziegler, "Adverse effects of cow's milk in infants." NCBI, 2007, , accessed September 30, 2017, https://www.ncbi.nlm.nih.gov/pubmed/17664905.

levels in males, as well as some cancers.[86, 87]

- Cow's milk is designed for growing calves (not humans) who begin their lives weighing 100 pounds and reach 800 pounds by the time they are weaned.

As you can see, feeding your child cow's milk may have more risks than benefits. Vitamin D3 and calcium are essential components of a growing baby's diet, but we can find them in sources that do not have added toxins such as cow's milk. Since vitamin D is naturally occurring in a limited number of foods (egg yolk, beef, and wild salmon, to name a few) and it is recommended by the American Academy of Pediatrics that your one-year-old receives 400 international units (IU) per day, you can administer vitamin D3 drops to your little one. Or if the sun is shining, taking your child for a walk (with most skin exposed and no sunblock) for around ten minutes will do the trick! Vitamin D and calcium complement each other with regard to the most efficient absorption of both nutrients, so for calcium intake, choose foods such as salmon, peas, broccoli, kale, collard greens, beans, oranges, and figs. Also, for a nutritious non-dairy beverage, try the following simple recipe for homemade nut milk.

Ingredients:

¾ cup raw almonds or cashews
2 cups filtered water
1 teaspoon honey or agave (optional)
Cinnamon to taste (optional)

Directions:

1. Soak the almonds for 8 hours, or the cashews for 3 hours.

2. Drain the nuts from the soaking water and place in a food processor or blender.

3. Blend the nuts while slowly adding filtered water until you have reached the desired consistency.

86 K. Maruyama, T. Oshima, and K. Ohyama, "Exposure to exogenous estrogen through intake of commercial milk produced from pregnant cows.," NCBI, February 2010, accessed September 20, 2017, https://www.ncbi.nlm.nih.gov/pubmed/19496976.
87 D. Ganmaa and A. Sato, "The possible role of female sex hormones in milk from pregnant cows in the development of breast, ovarian and corpus uteri cancers.," NCBI, 2005,, accessed September 30, 2017, https://www.ncbi.nlm.nih.gov/pubmed/16125328.

In addition to cow's milk, fruit juices have become a conventional beverage for babies and toddlers. Fruit juices do contain some essential vitamins but those vitamins come with a cost and that cost is an overabundance of sugar. On average, most one-year-olds should be consuming a maximum of 15 grams of sugar per day. As you can see by the following chart, just ½ cup of juice will come close to or exceed this daily maximum of sugar. Not to mention, conditioning an infant's or toddler's taste buds to expect sweet flavor when hydrating may lead to an aversion to plain water consumption, which will likely result in several servings of juice per day.

JUICE (½ Cup)	SUGAR (grams)
Orange	11 grams
Apple	12 grams
Cranberry	16 grams

Like most foods that are found on shelves and in packages, the processing of juice strips it of some nutrients that occur naturally in the whole fruit. We suggest feeding an actual orange, accompanied by water, to your child. This combination will hydrate and deliver fiber, calcium, and vitamin C with only a fraction of the sugar found in orange juice.

Nutrition for babies and toddlers can be complicated due to the amount of conflicting information out there, most of which has stemmed from the dollars spent on marketing campaigns of high profile baby food companies, so if you are overwhelmed or even surprised by the information found in this chapter and the previous one, you are not alone! By reading about baby's first solids, you have taken the first step in starting your child on a life-long path of good nutrition habits and excellent health!

Chapter 17
The Busy Mom's Meal Planning System

The Busy Mom's Meal Planning System is your simple guide to daily food recommendations that can be used during any and all trimesters of pregnancy. You may be wondering, *do I use the meal planning system or the recipes found in the following chapters?* The answer is both! The meal planning system found in this chapter is a road map of basic food choices to follow and it's specifically designed for women who don't have time for recipes. If you find yourself on a lazy Sunday where you do have some time to experiment, feel free to try the fancier breakfast, lunch, and dinner recipes found in the following three chapters.

Unlike the typical, rigid meal plan, the Buys Mom's Meal Planning System gives you several options for breakfast, lunch, dinner, beverages, and snacks—many are vegetarian and vegan-friendly as well! At the beginning of each section (breakfast, lunch, dinner, beverages, snacks), you will be given a set of directions which will explain possible food options for that particular meal or snack. This will allow for some flexibility with regard to your taste buds, how hungry you are, caloric needs based on your current trimester, and what you have in the pantry or refrigerator. The Busy Mom's Meal Planning System is based on simplicity, convenience, and foods that are sound with regard to prenatal nutrition. If you are feeling more adventurous, feel free to substitute any meal with one of the delicious recipes found in Chapters 18, 19, and 20. Or you can even create your own unique daily food plans using the breakfast, lunch, and dinner recipes found in those chapters as all meals exhibited provide dense nutrition for the expecting mom.

The items listed in the meal planning system are easily found in most grocery stores and the majority of the instructions (I won't even call them recipes) are simple, and do not call for too many ingredients or too much preparation. If you're unsure of the appropriate serving size, the nutrition label of a particular food will list how much of the item should be consumed for one serving, or you can refer to the serving size chart. Your caloric needs will differ based on the trimester of pregnancy you are currently in. Most normal weight women require the following but keep in mind, this is an average so your needs may be slightly less or slightly more.

TRIMESTER	Calories (Singleton)	Calories (Twins)	Calories (Triplets)
Trimester I	1800	2100	2250
Trimester II	2150	2480	2820
Trimester III	2250	2700	3150

Easy Serving Sizes

Serving of vegetables = a softball
Serving of fruit = a tennis ball
Serving of nuts or hummus = a golf ball
Serving of peanut or almond butter = a ping pong ball
Serving of green salad = a softball
Teaspoon of oil = a thumb
Serving of meat, poultry, or fish = 1½ decks of cards
Serving of cheese = four stacked dice
Serving of oatmeal or quinoa = a large fist
Serving of beans = small fist
Serving of yogurt or cottage cheese = a small fist

How to Meal Plan–Breakfast

Breakfast Directions: Choose one item each from both Category 1 and Category 2. If you only want one item total, choose it from either category. If choosing two items, do not make both selections from the same category.

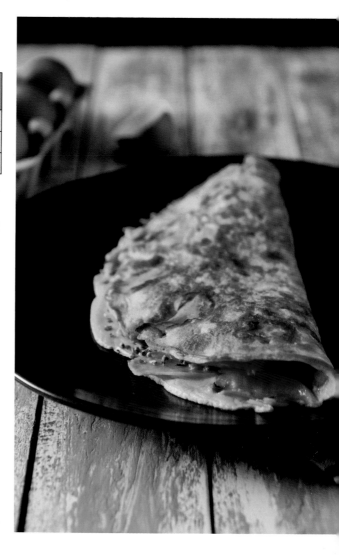

Category 1 Selections

Grapefruit: Slice a large grapefruit in half; save the other half for later.

Mixed Fruit: One small bowl of your favorite mixed fruits (not from a can).

Yogurt Parfait: Greek yogurt topped with berries of choice and crushed nuts; drizzle of honey or agave is optional.

Banana: One small banana.

Nut Butter Banana: One small banana dipped in real peanut or almond butter.

Cottage Cheese and Berries: Small bowl of cottage cheese topped with berries of choice.

Deluxe Oatmeal: Small bowl of oatmeal topped with almond or coconut milk, fruit of choice, and chia seeds; drizzle of honey or agave is optional.

Vegan Yogurt with Berries: Coconut or almond yogurt topped with berries of choice.

Vegan Banana Berry Protein Shake: Blend coconut or almond milk, blueberries, crushed walnuts, flaxseed meal, banana, and ice until smooth; add hemp powder for added protein and fiber (optional).

Green Vegan Protein Smoothie: Blend almond milk, avocado, kale, frozen banana, and chia seeds; add hemp powder for added protein and fiber (optional).

Category 2 Selections

One Egg Your Way: Choose your favorite preparation style—boiled, poached, scrambled, over-easy, or sunny-side up. When opting for scrambled, over-easy, or sunny-side up, use extra-virgin olive oil.

Two Eggs Your Way: Choose your favorite preparation style—boiled, poached, scrambled, over-easy, or sunny-side up. When opting for scrambled, over-easy, or sunny-side up, use extra-virgin olive oil.

Quick & Easy Scramble: Using extra-virgin olive and your favorite seasonings, sauté diced onions, diced bell peppers, and mushrooms in a pan for 5 minutes or until tender. In a separate bowl, scramble 2 eggs and then pour on top of the sautéed onions, bell peppers, and mushrooms. Cook through to your liking, gently folding and scrambling the eggs with the onions, bell peppers, and mushrooms. Sprinkle your favorite cheese on top (optional).

Breakfast Sandwich Scramble: Pan-cook 2 slices of nitrate-free bacon, chop, and add to a small bowl. Add 2 raw eggs to the same bowl and scramble. Using extra-virgin olive oil, pan-cook the egg/bacon mixture until cooked through. Top with grated cheddar cheese and sliced avocado.

Spinach and Cheese Omelet: Using extra-virgin olive oil and your favorite seasonings, sauté a handful of fresh spinach in a small pan for 5 minutes or until wilted down. In a separate bowl, beat 2 eggs together and then pour egg mixture on top of the spinach. Cook on low-medium heat for 3 minutes. Place your favorite cheese on top of the cooking egg mixture. Using a spatula, fold one half of your omelet over and cook for another 5 minutes or until cooked through to your liking.

Tempeh Scramble: Using extra-virgin olive oil and your favorite seasonings, sauté sliced onions and bell peppers for 5 minutes; add sliced mushrooms to the pan and cook for a few more minutes until everything is somewhat tender. Add crumbled tempeh and continue to cook for 3 minutes. Stir in halved cherry tomatoes and serve.

Protein Pancakes: Mash ripe banana with a fork and then thoroughly combine with 2 raw eggs until smooth, then add a dash of cinnamon. Pour silver-dollar-sized pancakes and cook in coconut or extra-virgin olive oil for 1 minute on one side

and 30 seconds on the other side; top with your favorite berries. *This meal provides a balance of carbohydrates, protein, and fat, so we do not recommend adding a selection from Category 1 if choosing this meal.*

Banana Nut Protein Pancakes: Mash 1 ripe banana with a fork and then thoroughly combine with 2 raw eggs and a dollop of almond or peanut butter until smooth. Cook in coconut or extra-virgin olive oil for 1 minute on one side and 30 seconds on the other side (silver-dollar-sized pancakes); top with your favorite berries. *This meal provides a balance of carbohydrates, protein, and fat so we do not recommend adding a selection from Category 1 if choosing this meal.*

Flaxseed Pancakes: Whisk 3 tablespoons ground flaxseed with 7 tablespoons water and sit aside in the refrigerator for 20 minutes to thicken. Mash ¾ of a large banana with a fork in a small mixing bowl and combine with the flaxseed/water mixture until you have a batter-like consistency. Using extra-virgin olive oil, cook your pancakes over medium heat until cooked through (2 minutes on each side). Top with cinnamon. *This meal provides a balance of carbohydrates,* *protein, and fat so we do not recommend adding a selection from Category 1 if choosing this meal.*

How to Meal Plan—Lunch

Lunch Directions: Choose one lunch meal. All items in the dinner section make for nutritionally acceptable lunches as well, but since many people do not have time to cook at lunch, some of the below meals are based on convenience, minimal preparation time (less than 15 minutes), the ability to make large quantities that will keep well in the refrigerator, and ease of transporting out of the house.

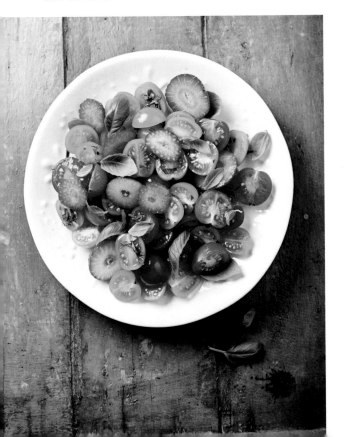

Snack Pack Meal: 1 hard-boiled egg, apple slices, raw cashews or raw almonds, Greek yogurt, and your favorite vegetables dipped in hummus.

Tuna Salad Snack Pack: Mix 1 can of chunk-light tuna with extra-virgin olive oil, diced celery, diced onion, diced tomato, diced avocado, black pepper, mustard, and lemon juice (use endive leaves or celery sticks to dip), one string cheese, and a handful of strawberries.

Vegan Snack Pack: Your favorite vegetables dipped in hummus, raw almonds or cashews, almond or coconut yogurt topped with your favorite berries.

Lettuce Wrap "Sandwiches": Fill large lettuce leaves with chunks of turkey or chicken breast, diced onion, diced tomato, avocado, and shredded cheese; top with black pepper and mustard.

Taco Lettuce Wrap "Sandwiches": Fill large lettuce leaves with chunks of chicken breast, black beans, dollop of Greek yogurt, salsa, sliced avocado, shredded cheese, and cilantro.

Vegan Taco Lettuce Wrap "Sandwiches": Fill large lettuce leaves with black beans or refried beans (make sure only ingredient is beans if buying canned), salsa, sliced avocado, and cilantro.

Lentil and Hummus Lettuce Wrap "Sandwiches": Mix cooked lentils with hummus in a small bowl. Fill large lettuce leaves with the mixture and top with diced cucumber, diced onion, diced tomato, and fresh parsley (optional).

Mayo-free Egg Salad Lettuce Wrap "Sandwiches": Dice two hard-boiled eggs and combine with two tablespoons hummus in a small bowl. Fill large lettuce leaves with the mixture and top with diced tomato and avocado.

Lettuce Wrap "Sandwiches" Your Way: Fill large lettuce leaves with your favorite sandwich items. Suggested: turkey breast, chicken breast, lean beef, canned tuna, canned salmon, fish, shrimp, tempeh, black beans, garbanzo beans, pinto beans, kidney beans, lentils, quinoa, tomato, avocado, onion, shredded cheese, Greek yogurt, red salsa, green salsa, extra virgin olive oil, balsamic vinegar, lemon, lime, and fresh herbs.

Protein-Packed Vegan Quinoa Salad: Cook red or white quinoa according to package, and toss with diced tomatoes, diced red onions, diced cucumber, parsley, cilantro, extra-virgin olive oil, apple cider vinegar, and freshly squeezed lemon juice.

Protein Packed Vegan Greens and Bean Salad: In a large bowl, combine mixed greens, sprouts, diced tomatoes, red onion, avocado, broccoli florets, kidney beans, garbanzo beans, and pinto beans. Thoroughly toss with extra-virgin olive oil, freshly squeezed lemon juice, and balsamic vinegar.

Vegan Bean Trio Salad: Toss your favorite trio of beans (our favorite combination is garbanzo, kidney, and black beans) and thinly sliced green onion with extra-virgin olive oil, apple cider vinegar, garlic, lime juice, honey, ginger, and pepper.

Mexican Platter: Pan-cook cubed boneless skinless chicken breasts with extra-virgin olive oil and favorite low-sodium taco seasoning. Plate with a side of black beans topped with shredded cheese, side of shredded lettuce or cabbage, dollop of Greek yogurt, salsa, sliced avocado, and cilantro.

The Works Salad: Mixed greens topped with your favorite protein (chicken, fish, shellfish, canned tuna, turkey, lean beef), diced tomatoes, diced onions, avocado, and shredded cheese. Top with extra-virgin olive oil and balsamic vinegar.

Protein Soup and Salad: Your favorite high protein soup (suggestions are split pea, lentil, black bean, vegetable beef, and chicken and vegetable) paired with mixed green salad topped with your favorite salad dressing (see Chapter 21 for salad dressing recipes).

Guilt-Free Spaghetti: Cut a whole spaghetti squash in half, scoop out stringy pieces and seeds, and place halves face down on a baking sheet and bake at 400° F for 35–50 minutes or until tender. Using a fork, shred the flesh of the cooked squash into "noodles" and top with your favorite spaghetti sauce and grated Parmesan cheese.

Turkey Burger: Grill or pan-cook ground turkey burger with extra-virgin olive oil and your favorite seasonings. Top with a slice of your favorite cheese, lettuce leaves, sliced tomato, avocado, and mustard.

High Protein Lentil Salad: Mix already cooked and chilled lentils (you can buy them this way to save time) with dried cranberries, parsley, fresh mint, and diced cucumber; top with a dollop of Greek yogurt.

Simple Protein and Vegetables: Your favorite lean protein paired with your choice of green vegetables.

How to Meal Plan—Dinner

Dinner Directions: Choose up to two items from Category 1 (at least one selection must be green) *or* choose one item from Category 1 (must be green) *and* one item from Category 3. Also choose one item from Category 2 (non-vegan proteins) *or* one item from Category 3 (vegan proteins).

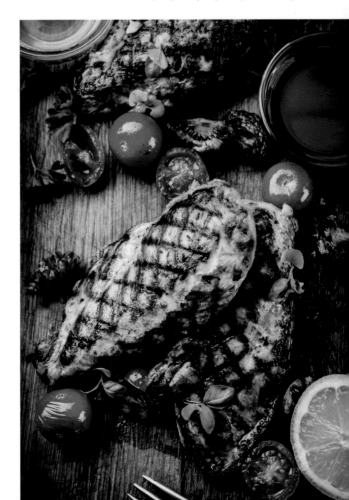

Category 1 Selections

Grilled Asparagus: Toss asparagus in extra-virgin olive oil, garlic, and black pepper; grill on BBQ or in pan until tender; top with freshly squeezed lemon juice.

Sautéed Brussels Sprouts: Slice Brussels sprouts in half and remove stem. Pan-sauté with extra-virgin olive oil, garlic, black pepper, and minced onion (optional) until tender; top with freshly squeezed lemon juice.

Fancy Mixed Greens Salad: Mixed greens of choice tossed with dried cranberries, diced red onions, crushed walnuts, diced tomatoes, goat cheese, and sliced avocado. Top with your favorite salad dressing (see Chapter 21).

Simple Mixed Greens: Mixed greens of choice tossed with diced onions and tomatoes; top with extra-virgin olive oil and balsamic vinegar.

Caprese Salad: 2 thick slices of tomato topped with 2 slices of Mozzarella, basil leaves, extra-virgin olive oil, and balsamic vinegar.

Fennel Citrus Salad: Thinly slice a bulb of fennel and plate with slices or chunks of orange, grapefruit, and avocado. For the dressing, combine extra-virgin olive oil with sherry vinegar, fresh lemon juice, and a drizzle of honey; toss thoroughly through the salad.

Mashed Cauliflower: Steam and mash 1 head of cauliflower (just like you do with potatoes) and combine with 3 tablespoons of grated Parmesan cheese.

Riced Cauliflower: Steam 1 head of cauliflower until tender; use a fork to shred the cauliflower into a rice-like texture.

Sautéed Kale: Chop kale leaves in 2 x 2-inch squares (some grocery stores sell it already chopped) and pan-sauté over low-medium heat with extra-virgin olive oil, minced onion, and minced garlic until tender (around 5–7 minutes); top with fresh lemon juice.

Steamed Broccoli: Steam broccoli until tender; top with freshly squeezed lemon juice and black pepper.

Baked Broccoli: Toss broccoli florets with extra-virgin olive oil, garlic, and herbs of choice. Bake until tender (around 25 minutes) at 350° F. Top with grated Parmesan and freshly squeezed lemon juice.

Grilled Romaine Salad: Slice head of romaine in half lengthwise. Spray both sides of lettuce head halves with extra-virgin olive oil. Grill for 2 minutes on each side and top with grated Parmesan.

Roasted Fennel: Remove the stem of the fennel (only the bulb is used for this dish); slice the bulb into quarters, and steam for 15 minutes or until moderately tender. Toss in extra-virgin olive oil. Roast at 375°F for 10 minutes; top with grated Parmesan when there are 2 minutes left.

Roasted Mixed Vegetables: Toss carrot pieces, cauliflower florets, and broccoli florets with extra-virgin olive oil and bake in pan at 350°F until tender (around 25 minutes). Top with grated Parmesan and freshly squeezed lemon juice.

Sautéed Butternut Squash and Apples: Cut butternut squash and apples into small cubes (you can buy already chopped butternut squash at some stores) and pan-sauté with extra-virgin olive oil and sage until tender.

Roasted Fingerling Potatoes: Toss with extra-virgin olive oil and your favorite seasonings; roast for 20 minutes at 425°F.

Baked Sweet Potato: Pierce the sweet potato 5 times with a fork and bake on a foil-lined baking sheet for 45 minutes to an hour, or until tender.

Category 2 Selections (Non-vegan)

Boneless and skinless chicken breasts	Ground beef
Ground chicken	Wild salmon
Boneless and skinless chicken tenders	Cod
Turkey breast cutlets	Halibut
Ground turkey	Rockfish
Pork chops	Sole
Grass-fed beef	Prawns/Shrimp
Lamb chops	Scallops
Bison	Crab
Venison	

Preparation Style: Choose a preparation style for your protein.

Grilled: Lightly coat your protein with extra-virgin olive oil and your favorite herbs (see add-ons/condiments chapter for suggestions). Grill on both sides until cooked through to your liking. Top with freshly squeezed lemon juice for added flavor.

Pan-cooked: Put 1–2 tablespoons (based on the servings of food you are preparing) of extra-virgin olive oil in a pan. Add your favorite herbs and seasonings to the oil. Pan-cook on medium-high heat until lightly browned on each side; reduce heat to medium-low until cooked through to your liking.

Baked: Lightly coat your protein with extra-virgin olive oil and favorite herbs and seasonings. Bake at 350–400°F (depends on the protein) until cooked through to your liking. For added flavor (optional), dress up your protein with your favorite sauce (see Chapter 21 for sauce recipes).

Sautéed: Pan-sauté your protein over low-medium heat in your favorite sauce/ marinade (see Chapter 21 for sauce recipes).

Category 3 Selections (Vegan)

Quinoa	Navy Beans
Lentils	Mixed Beans
Black Beans	Peas
Garbanzo Beans	Tempeh
Lima Beans	Natto
Pinto Beans	Cooked Spinach

Snacks

Directions: Choose 1 or 2 snacks per day to eat between meals. For more snack recipes and ideas, refer to Chapter 21.

One serving of your favorite fruit
½ apple dipped in real peanut or almond butter
Celery dipped in real peanut or almond butter
Handful of raw nuts or seeds
Your favorite vegetables dipped in hummus
Your favorite vegetables dipped in mashed avocado
Hard-boiled egg
One piece of cheese
One serving Greek yogurt
One serving coconut or almond yogurt
One serving of lentils, peas, or beans
Small side salad

Condiments and Add-Ons

Directions: Use any of the following condiments or add-ons to put your own spin on a meal, snack, or beverage.

salsa	chia seeds
pico De Gallo	flaxseeds
green tomatillo sauce	raw nuts
mustard	extra-virgin olive oil
lettuce	coconut oil
tomato	avocado oil
onion	grapeseed oil
shallots	apple cider vinegar
bell pepper	balsamic vinegar
avocado	gluten-free vinegar of choice
mushroom	hot sauce
grated cheese	tamari
Greek yogurt	tahini
hummus	parsley
drizzle of honey	cilantro
drizzle of agave	tarragon
garlic	mint
ginger	rosemary
Parmesan cheese	thyme
freshly squeezed lemon juice	black pepper
freshly squeezed lime juice	turmeric
sunflower seeds	cinnamon
hemp seeds	your favorite herbs/spices.

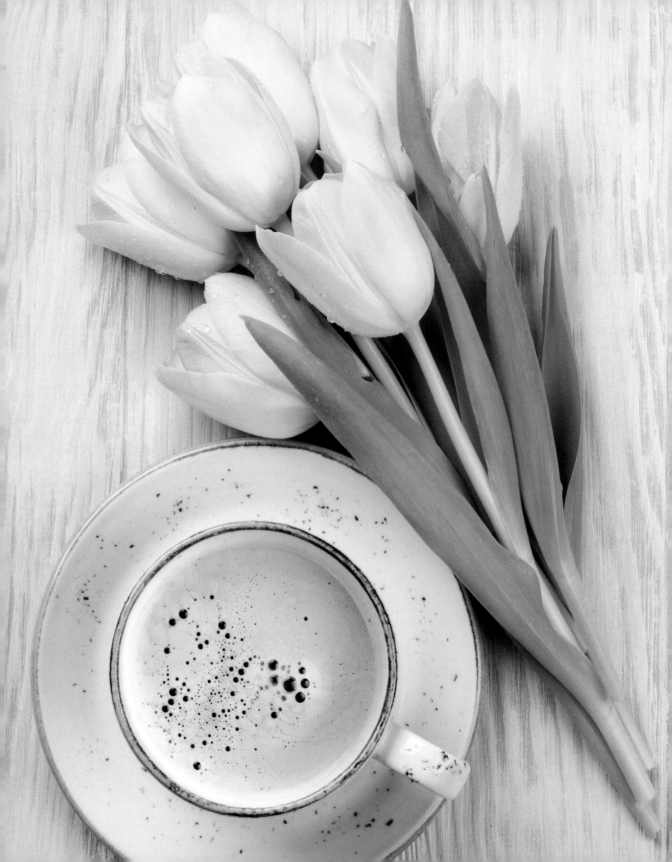

Chapter 18
The Whole Food Pregnancy
Breakfast Recipes

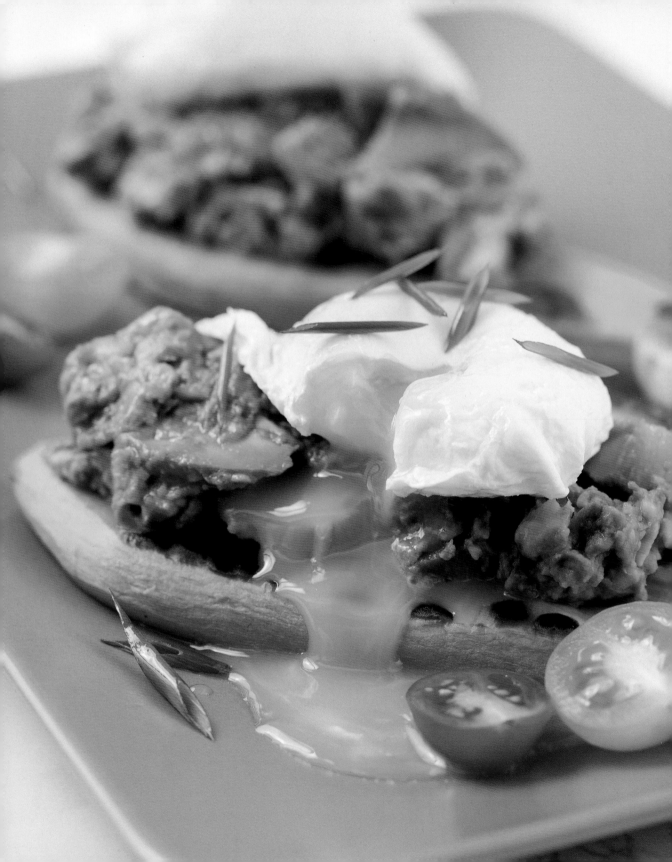

Avocado Sweet Potato "Toast"

serves 3

Ingredients:

1 large sweet potato, sliced into ½-inch planks
1 tablespoon extra-virgin olive oil
Your favorite seasonings
1 avocado, mashed
3 whole eggs
Grape tomatoes, halved, and chives for garnish (optional)

For vegan option, replace eggs with sprouts and sliced radishes.

Directions:

1. Preheat oven to 450° F.

2. Slice off 4 rounded sides of the sweet potato so it sits flat on cutting board; proceed to slice the sweet potatoes into three ½-inch planks.

3. Toss the sweet potato planks in extra-virgin olive oil and your favorite seasonings; place on baking sheet.

4. Roast for 15 minutes or until lightly browned and tender, flipping over halfway through.

5. Meanwhile, mash the avocado in a bowl, leaving some small chunks.

6. When sweet potatoes are 5–7 minutes away from being done, prepare poached or sunny-side up eggs.

7. When sweet potatoes are finished roasting, plate them and top each plank with avocado mash and 1 egg (replace egg with sprouts and sliced radish for vegan option).

8. Garnish with halved grape tomatoes and chives (optional).

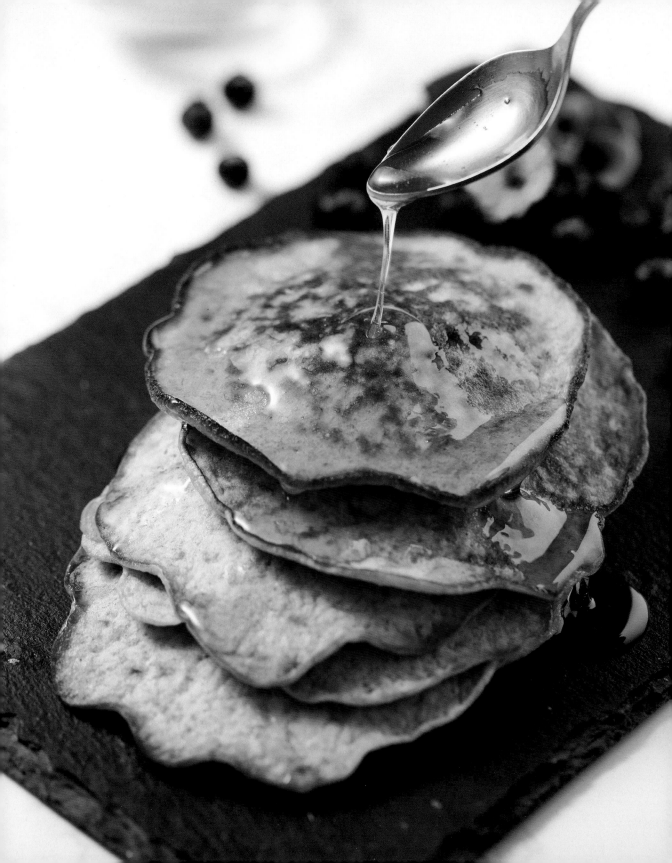

Three-Ingredient Protein Pancake

serves 1

Ingredients:

1 ripe banana
2 whole eggs
1 teaspoon extra-virgin olive oil
Ground cinnamon to taste

Directions:

1. Using a fork, mash the banana into a creamy texture (small lumps okay).

2. Add the eggs and combine until smooth.

3. Using extra-virgin olive oil, pan-cook just as you would with regular pancake batter (flip the pancake after 2 minutes of cooking over medium heat or until batter begins to change from liquid to a firm consistency).

4. Cook for 1 minute after the pancake has been flipped; remove from heat immediately.

5. Top with ground cinnamon.

Papaya-Ginger Smoothie

serves 1

Ingredients:

2½ cups papaya chunks (refrigerated)
1 cup ice cubes
⅔ cup Greek yogurt (substitute coconut or almond yogurt for vegan option)

1 tablespoon finely chopped peeled fresh ginger
1 tablespoon honey
Juice of 2 lemons
16 fresh mint leaves

Directions:

1. Blend papaya, ice, yogurt, ginger, honey, and lemon juice in a blender or food processor.

2. Add one or two tablespoons of water until you have reached desired consistency.

3. Blend in mint leaves.

High Protein Quinoa Oatmeal

serves 1

Ingredients:

¼ cup water
2 egg whites
¼ cup dry quinoa
1 teaspoon chia seeds
1 teaspoon ground flax seeds
1 tablespoon fresh pomegranate seeds (optional)
Handful of fresh raspberries (optional)

Directions:

1. Whisk water and egg whites together in a small pot.

2. Add dry quinoa and stir over medium heat until cooked through to your desired tenderness and texture (about 15 minutes).

3. Top with chia and flax seeds and fresh berries.

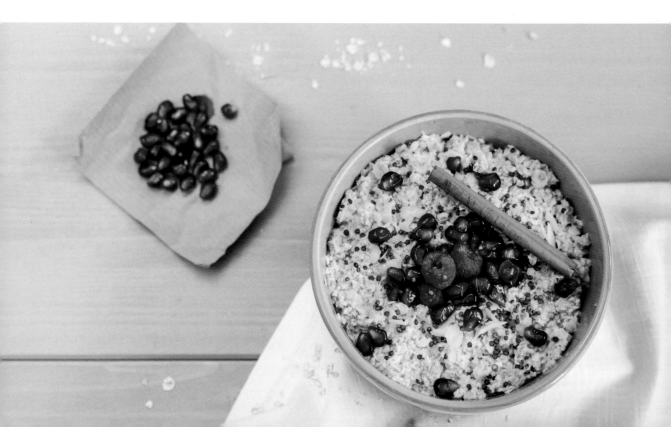

Almond Coconut Breakfast Quinoa

serves 3-4

Ingredients:

1 cup quinoa
1 cup water
1 cup coconut milk
2 tablespoons maple syrup (optional)
½ cup chopped or slivered almonds
½ cup shredded, unsweetened coconut
Almond milk (for topping)

Directions:

1. Place quinoa in medium saucepan with water and coconut milk over medium-high heat.

2. Bring to light boil while stirring; change to heat to low, cover and let simmer for 10–15 minutes while stirring occasionally.

3. Remove from heat and allow to sit for 5 minutes.

4. Add maple syrup, almonds, coconut, and almond milk to desired consistency.

Lactation Breakfast Shake
(great for non-nursing mothers too!)

serves 1

Ingredients:

½ cup coconut water
½ cup almond milk
1 banana
1 cup ice

¼ cup gluten-free dry oats (steel cut or regular)
1 dollop of peanut or almond butter
1 tablespoon gluten-free brewer's yeast (optional)

Directions:

1. Using a blender, combine all ingredients until desired consistency.

Kale and Red Pepper Frittata

serves 4

Ingredients:

8 large eggs

½ cup almond or coconut milk

Your favorite seasonings to taste

1 tablespoon extra-virgin olive oil

½ cup chopped red bell pepper

⅓ cup chopped onion

2 cups chopped kale, rinsed with stems removed

Directions:

1. Preheat oven to 350° F.
2. Whisk the eggs and milk together and add your favorite seasonings. Set aside.
3. In a skillet, heat extra-virgin olive oil over medium heat. Add onion and red pepper and sauté for 3 minutes, until onion is tender. Add kale and cook for 5 minutes or until kale is wilted.
4. Add eggs to the pan mixture and cook for about 4 minutes until the bottom and edges of the frittata start to set.
5. Put frittata in the oven and cook for 10–15 minutes until the frittata is cooked all the way through. Slice and serve.

Sweet Potato Hash and Eggs

serves 1–2

Ingredients:

1 tablespoon extra-virgin olive oil

1 small sweet potato, cubed

½ small yellow onion, chopped

½ bell pepper, chopped

Your favorite seasonings

2 tablespoons of cilantro or parsley, chopped

2 whole eggs

Half an avocado, diced

Directions:

1. In a small pan over medium heat, cook the potatoes, onions, and bell pepper with extra-virgin olive oil and your favorite seasonings; leave covered for 5–7 minutes or until softened.
2. Remove lid and cook for another 2–3 minutes until browned.
3. Add the cilantro or parsley (or both if you prefer) and cook for another 2–3 minutes.
4. Top with two pan-cooked or poached eggs.
5. Garnish with avocado and more cilantro or parsley.

Greek Yogurt Parfait

serves 1

Ingredients:

½ cup Greek yogurt

Handful of your favorite berries

Handful of crushed walnuts

1 teaspoon chia seeds

Drizzle of honey or agave (optional)

Directions:

1. Place the Greek yogurt in a bowl.

2. Top with berries, walnuts, chia seeds, and honey or agave.

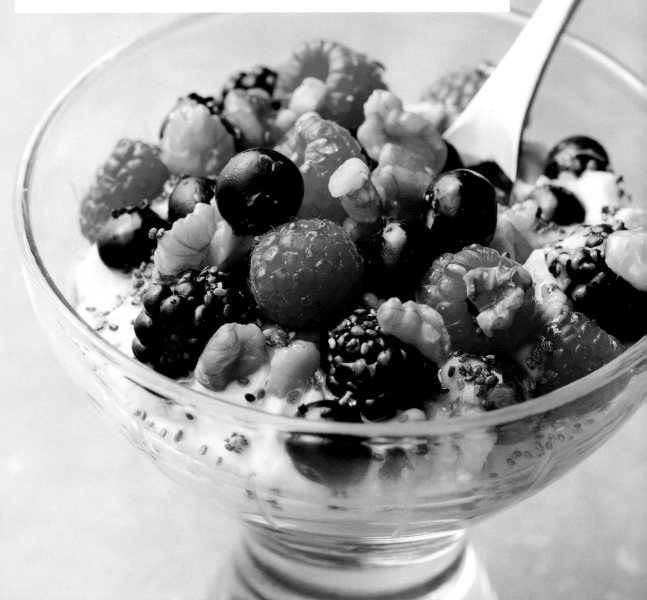

Ginger-Coconut Chia Seed Breakfast Pudding

serves 1

Ingredients:

½ banana

¼ cup unsweetened coconut milk

3 ounces 2% or whole Greek yogurt (optional for added protein—the chia seeds will thicken the yogurt on their own)

1 tablespoon chia seeds

1 teaspoon freshly grated ginger

Fresh berries (optional)

Directions:

1. Mash the banana and then whisk with coconut milk and Greek yogurt.

2. Stir in the chia seeds and ginger and refrigerate for two hours or until the pudding thickens.

3. Top with your favorite berries (optional).

Easy Cheesy Vegetable Scramble

serves 1

Ingredients:

1 tablespoon extra-virgin olive oil

½ cup chopped onion, bell pepper, and mushroom (the mixture should total ½ cup)

2 whole eggs

1 slice of your favorite cheese, chopped

½ avocado, sliced

Directions:

1. Sauté the chopped onion, bell pepper, and mushroom in extra-virgin olive oil over medium heat for 5 minutes or until all ingredients are tender.

2. Scramble eggs in a small bowl and add the chopped cheese; combine.

3. Add scrambled egg and cheese mixture to pan and cook until eggs are at desired temperature.

4. Top with sliced avocado (optional).

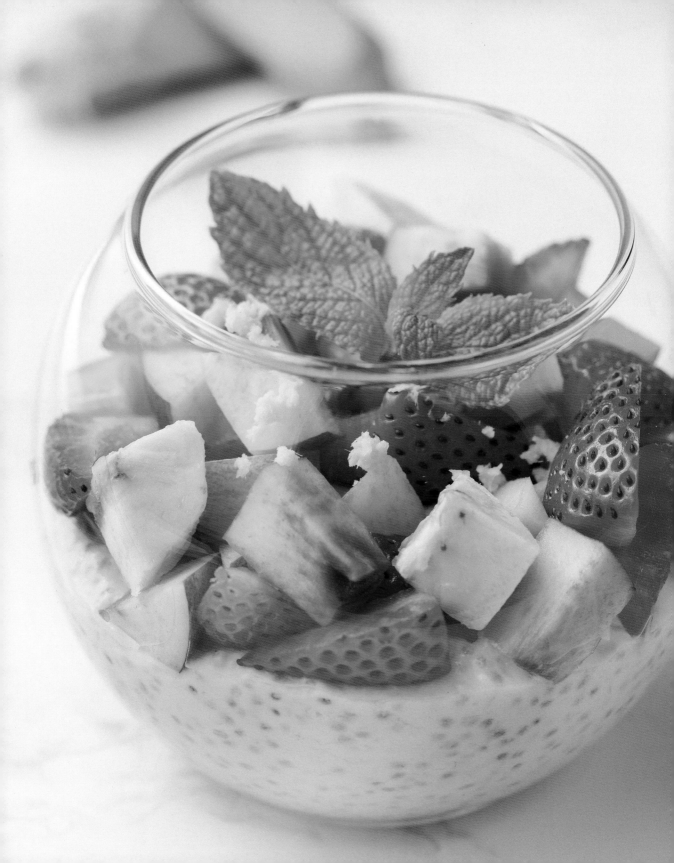

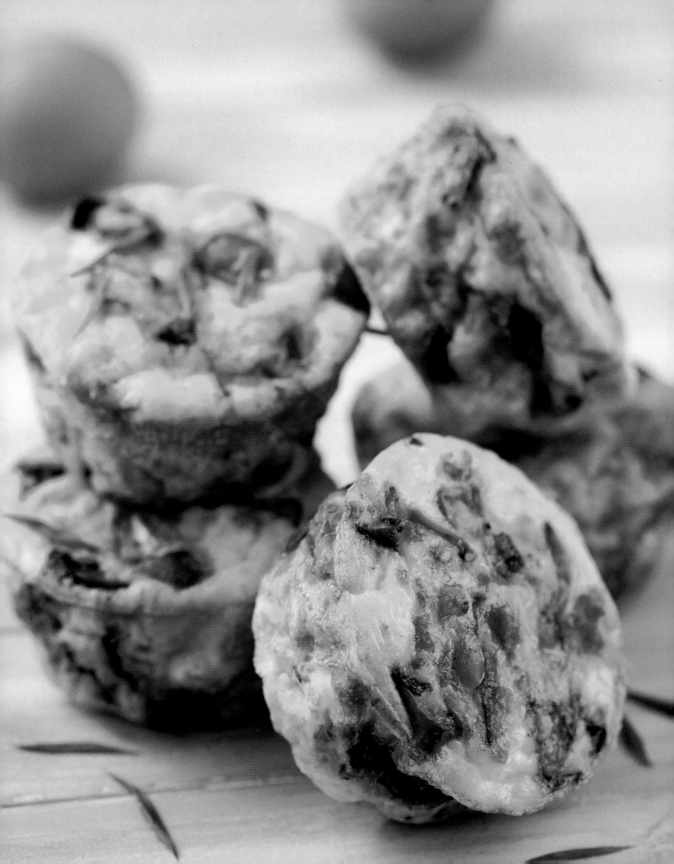

Egg "Muffins"

makes 10 muffins

Ingredients:

1–2 tablespoons extra-virgin olive oil
1 large Portobello mushroom, diced
2 handfuls of fresh spinach
1 small onion, diced
1 red or orange bell pepper, diced
½ cup cooked and crumbled turkey or lean ground beef (optional)
8 whole eggs
Your favorite seasonings to taste
½ cup grated fresh Parmesan cheese

Directions:

1. Preheat oven to 350° F.

2. Heat 1 tablespoon extra-virgin olive oil over medium heat and sauté the mushrooms, spinach, onion, and pepper for 5 minutes. Season to taste and add more extra-virgin olive oil if needed.

3. Spoon the sautéed vegetables into individual muffin slots on standard muffin pan.

4. If using, pan-cook your meat of choice and divide equally between muffin slots.

5. In a separate bowl, whisk together the eggs and season to taste with preferred seasonings.

6. Pour egg mixture into each muffin slot and mix in with the vegetables and meat.

7. Evenly sprinkle the tops of each muffin with the Parmesan cheese.

8. Bake for 14–16 minutes until the eggs are completely set.

Breakfast Burrito Bowl

serves 2

Ingredients:

1 tablespoon extra-virgin olive oil
1 small potato, finely chopped
¼ cup white onion, diced
¼ cup bell pepper, diced
½ cup black beans
3 whole eggs, scrambled
2 strips nitrate-free bacon, cooked and diced (optional)
¼ cup cheddar cheese, grated
1 tablespoon Greek yogurt or sour cream
Mild salsa to taste

Directions:

1. Using extra-virgin olive oil, pan-sauté the potato, onion, and bell pepper until tender. Meanwhile, place beans in a medium bowl.

3. Add the raw scrambled eggs to the pan mixture and cook on low-medium heat until the eggs are cooked through.

4. Combine with the previously cooked bacon and top with grated cheese; place the cooked egg mixture on top of the beans.

5. Garnish with Greek yogurt and salsa.

Breakfast "Granola" Bars

makes 6–8 bars

Ingredients:

¾ cup raw almonds
¾ cup macadamia nuts
¼ cup pumpkin seeds
¼ cup sunflower seeds
¼ cup unsweetened shredded coconut
½ cup dried cranberries or currants
½ cup melted coconut oil
¼ cup honey or real maple syrup
2 eggs
2 tablespoons cinnamon

Directions:

1. Preheat your oven to 400° F.

2. Place almonds and macadamia nuts in a food processor and pulse until you have a chunky mixture (avoid a flour-like texture).

3. Transfer the mixture to a large mixing bowl and add all other ingredients.

4. Mix well by hand to combine all ingredients thoroughly.

5. Grease a 9×9-inch square baking dish with coconut oil and then transfer your nut mixture to the dish.

6. Bake for 20–25 minutes; insert a toothpick at minute 20 to see if the bars are cooked through (if so, the toothpick will be clean).

7. Remove from the oven and allow to cool and then place in refrigerator for at least 1 hour.

8. Remove from the fridge and then slice into bars the size of your choice; wrap bars in plastic and refrigerate for up to a week.

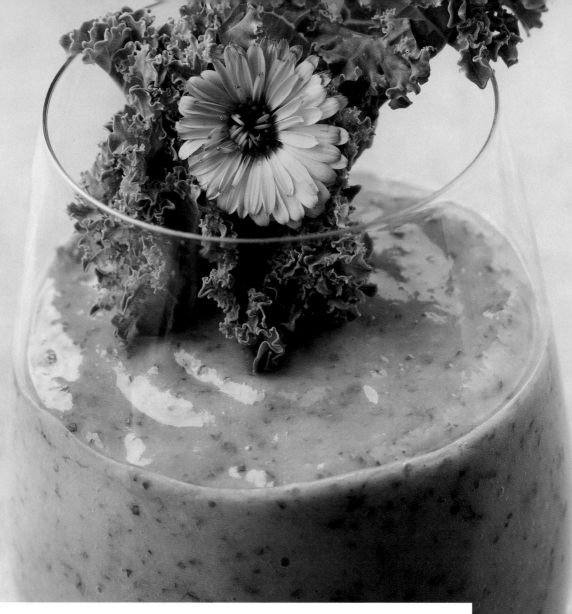

Banana Avocado Kale Smoothie

serves 1

Ingredients:

1 small banana (very ripe)

½ an avocado

½ cup kefir (milk or almond milk works too)

Handful of chopped kale

Handful of ice cubes

Directions:

1. Place all ingredients in a blender and blend until smooth.

Breakfast Casserole

serves 4

Ingredients:

6 ounces mozzarella cheese, shredded
6 ounces Colby-Monterey Jack cheese, shredded
1 tablespoon extra-virgin olive oil
6 ounces mushrooms, sliced
⅓ cup chopped green onion
½ medium red bell pepper, chopped
Large handful of fresh spinach leaves
½ cup almond flour
1¾ cups almond milk
2 tablespoons fresh parsley, chopped
8 eggs, beaten

Directions:

1. Preheat oven to 350° F.

2. Place cheeses in a large bowl and toss to combine.

3. Place half of the cheese blend on the bottom of a 9x13-inch casserole dish and spread evenly.

4. In a medium skillet, add extra-virgin olive oil, mushrooms, green onions, and peppers; cook until onion and pepper are tender.

5. Add in spinach leaves and cook for 2–3 minutes or until spinach is wilted.

6. Arrange cooked vegetables over cheese evenly.

7. In a large bowl whisk almond flour, milk, parsley, and eggs; pour on top of the vegetable and cheese layers.

8. Bake for 45 minutes or until set and lightly brown (with 5 minutes left of baking time, top casserole with the remaining cheese).

9. Cut into squares.

Refrigerator Oatmeal

serves 1

Ingredients:

⅓ cup almond milk

¼ cup gluten-free oats

¼ cup Greek yogurt

1 teaspoon honey or agave

Handful raw nuts of choice

1 teaspoon ground cinnamon

¼ cup fresh berries or fruit of choice

Directions:

1. Combine milk, oats, Greek yogurt, honey, nuts, and cinnamon in a small jar with a lid; cover, and shake until combined.

2. Remove lid and fold in berries; cover jar with lid.

3. Refrigerate oatmeal for 8 hours or overnight.

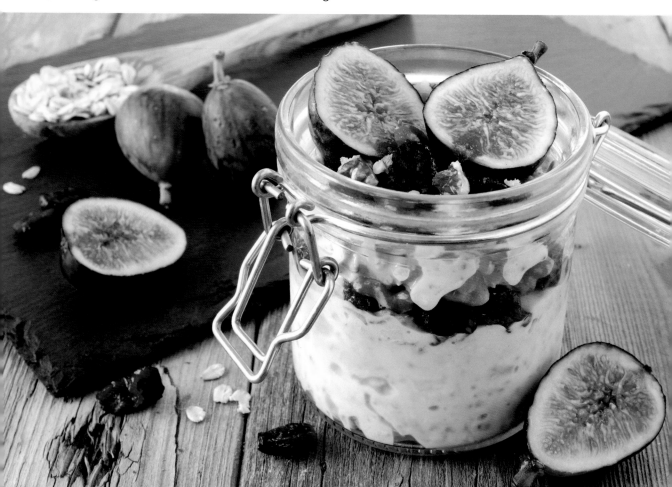

Sweet Potato Oatmeal

serves 2–3

Ingredients:

1 medium sweet potato

1 cup gluten-free oats

1 cup water (you may need a little more than these based on texture preferences)

½ cup unsweetened almond or coconut milk

Maple syrup to taste

1 teaspoon cinnamon

Dash nutmeg

1 tablespoon chia or ground flaxseeds (optional)

¼ cup chopped pecans or walnuts (optional)

Directions:

1. Using a fork, poke holes in a few places on the sweet potato and then roast for one hour at 400° F. If time does not permit, do this ahead of time and refrigerate your roasted sweet potato or cook in the microwave for 5–7 minutes.

2. When the sweet potato is almost done roasting, mix oatmeal with water in a small pot over medium heat until cooked through, adding more water if needed for desired consistency.

3. Cut open the roasted sweet potato and scoop out the insides. Combine the sweet potato and cooked oats until smooth.

4. Add remaining ingredients and toppings.

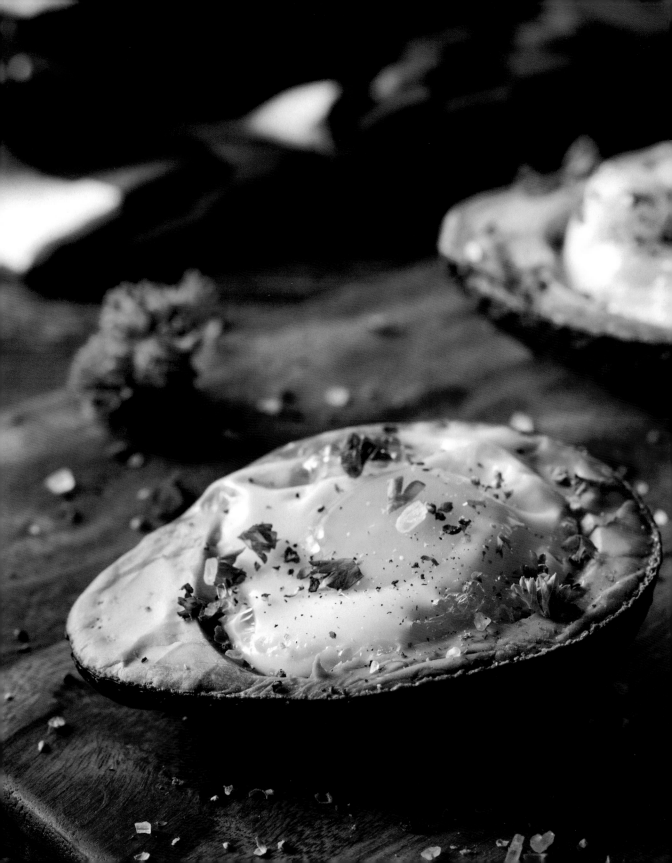

Loaded Baked Avocado

serves 1–2

Ingredients:

1 avocado, halved and pitted

2 whole eggs

Fresh lime wedge

Sprinkle of your favorite cheese (optional)

Chopped cilantro and scallions to taste

Dollop of Greek yogurt (optional)

Directions:

1. Preheat oven to 450° F.

2. Using a spoon, scrape out the center of each halved avocado so that it is large enough to accommodate an egg (about 1½ tablespoons).

3. Squeeze lime juice over the avocados and then place on baking sheet. Break an egg into the center of each avocado.

4. Bake for 10-12 minutes until whites are set and yolk is runny.

5. Add shredded cheese and continue to bake for 3 minutes. (If you do not top with cheese, continue to bake for 3 minutes without added cheese.)

6. Remove from oven and garnish with cilantro, scallions, and a dollop of Greek yogurt (optional).

Salmon Frittata

serves 3–4

Ingredients:

1 green bell pepper, chopped

1 onion, chopped

2 garlic cloves, minced

1 tablespoon extra-virgin olive oil

1 teaspoon cumin

½ teaspoon paprika

Sea salt and pepper to taste

1½ cups cherry tomatoes, halved

½ cup wild canned salmon

6 eggs beaten

2 tablespoons chopped cilantro

Directions:

1. Preheat the oven to 350° F.

2. Heat the oil in an oven-safe skillet over medium heat.

3. Pan-cook the pepper and onion for 5–6 minutes then add garlic and spices.

4. Once tender, add in the halved tomatoes.

5. Once tomatoes have softened, distribute the salmon evenly over the mixture.

6. Evenly pour the beaten eggs into the skillet so that everything is covered by the eggs.

7. Transfer the pan to the oven and cook for 15 minutes or until the eggs are set.

8. Remove from the oven and top with fresh cilantro.

Vegan Tempeh Hash

serves 4–6

Ingredients:

1 pound fingerling potatoes
2 tablespoons extra-virgin olive oil
1 medium onion, chopped
1 medium green or red bell pepper, diced
8-ounce package tempeh, diced
1 teaspoon paprika
6 leaves curly kale, stemmed and finely chopped
Salt and pepper to taste
Your favorite hot sauce (optional)

Directions:

1. Preheat oven to 500° F.

2. Wash and dry potatoes and then toss in half the extra-virgin olive oil.

3. Arrange them on a baking sheet in a single layer and place in oven; reduce heat to 425°, and roast for 20 minutes or until tender; after the potatoes have cooled, chop into small chunks.

4. Heat extra-virgin oil in a large skillet or pan. Add the onion and bell pepper and sauté over medium heat until tender.

5. Add the tempeh and potatoes; turn the heat up to medium-high, and continue to sauté (while stirring frequently) until it all turns golden brown.

6. Add the seasonings and kale and continue cooking for 3 more minutes; gradually add small amounts of water if the mixture gets too dry.

7. Season with salt and pepper and garnish with freshly chopped cilantro and hot sauce (optional).

Apple Cinnamon Oatmeal Muffins

makes 6 muffins

Ingredients:

Coconut oil for greasing
1 cup gluten-free rolled oats
1 whole egg
½ cup unsweetened applesauce
2 tablespoons honey, agave, or pure maple syrup
1 tablespoon cinnamon and a little extra for dusting
2 tablespoons unsweetened coconut
½ an apple, diced

Directions:

1. Preheat oven to 180° F. Lightly grease a muffin tin with coconut oil.

2. Blend together all ingredients except apple and coconut.

3. Pour muffin mix into greased muffin tin.

4. Top each muffin with unsweetened coconut, apple, and cinnamon.

5. Bake for 22 minutes (or until toothpick comes out clean).

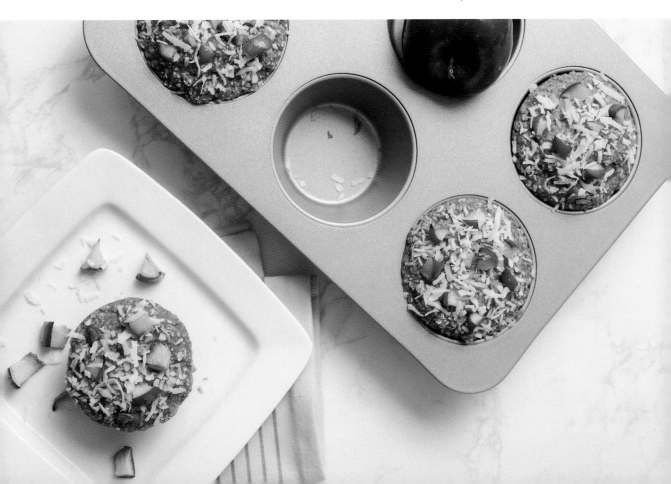

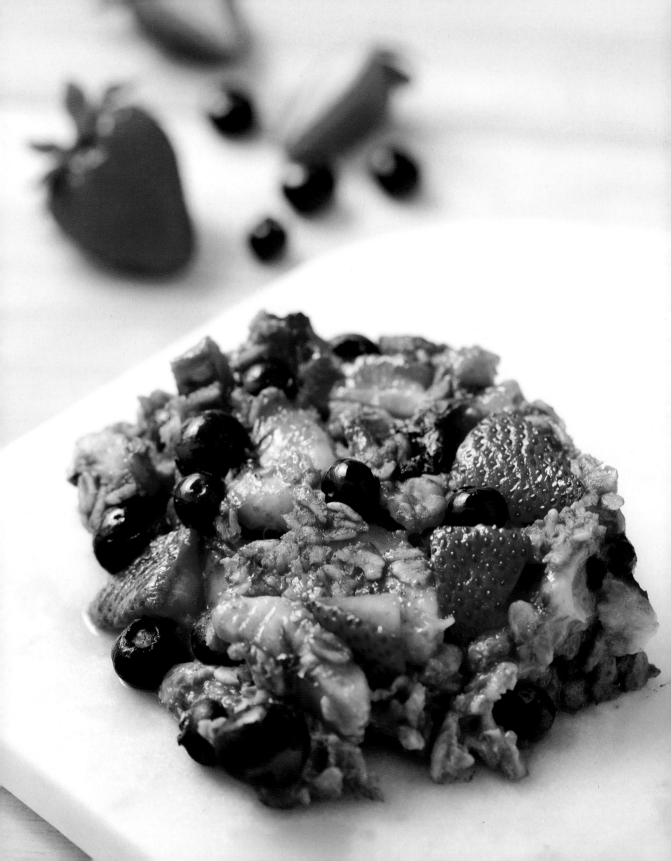

Baked Banana Berry Oatmeal

makes 6–8 squares

Ingredients:

2 ripe bananas, sliced into ½-inch pieces
1½ cup blueberries
1 cup strawberries, sliced
¼ cup honey or agave
1 cup gluten-free, uncooked rolled oats
¼ cup chopped pecans or walnuts
1 teaspoon cinnamon
1 cup almond or coconut milk
1 egg
1 teaspoon vanilla extract

Directions:

1. Preheat the oven to 375° F.

2. Lightly spray an 8 x 8" or 9 x 9" baking dish with extra-virgin olive oil or use coconut oil to lightly grease. Set aside.

3. Thoroughly combine all ingredients. Pour into your prepared dish.

4. Bake the oatmeal for about 30 minutes, or until the top is golden brown and the oatmeal has set.

5. Serve warm from the oven or refrigerate and cut into squares.

Cheesy Cauliflower Hash Browns & Eggs

serves 1

Ingredients:

¼ head cauliflower
½ cup cheddar cheese, grated
2 large eggs
½ cup almond flour
Your favorite seasonings
1 tablespoon extra-virgin olive oil

Directions:

1. Cut cauliflower into florets and steam until tender (around 15–20 minutes).

2. Drain and mash the cauliflower while still warm (just as you would do with potatoes).

3. Stir in cheese, eggs, almond flour, and seasonings.

4. Lightly coat the bottom of a griddle or skillet with extra-virgin olive oil over medium-high heat.

5. Form the cauliflower mixture into patties that are about 3 inches across and cook on each side until golden brown (about 3 minutes per side).

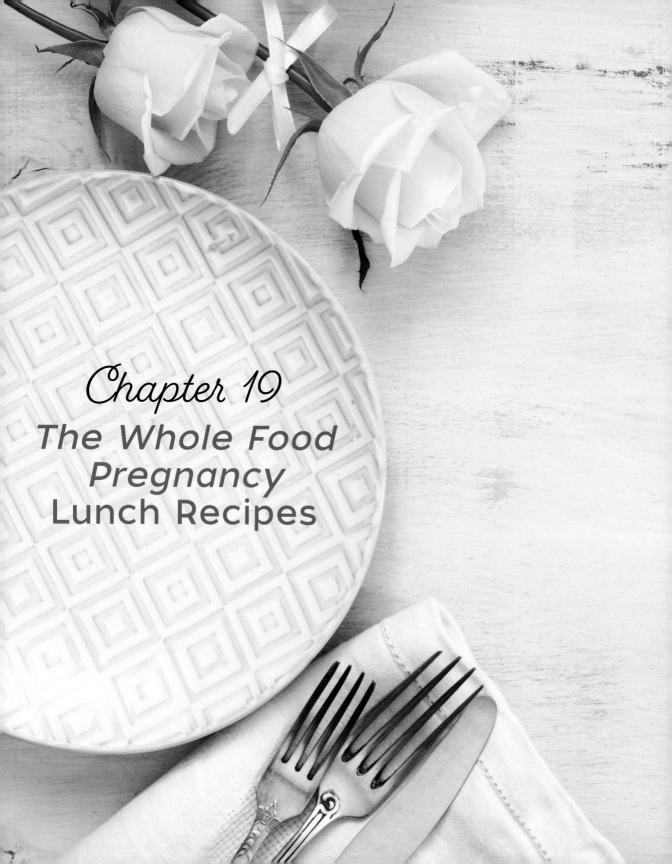

Chapter 19
The Whole Food Pregnancy Lunch Recipes

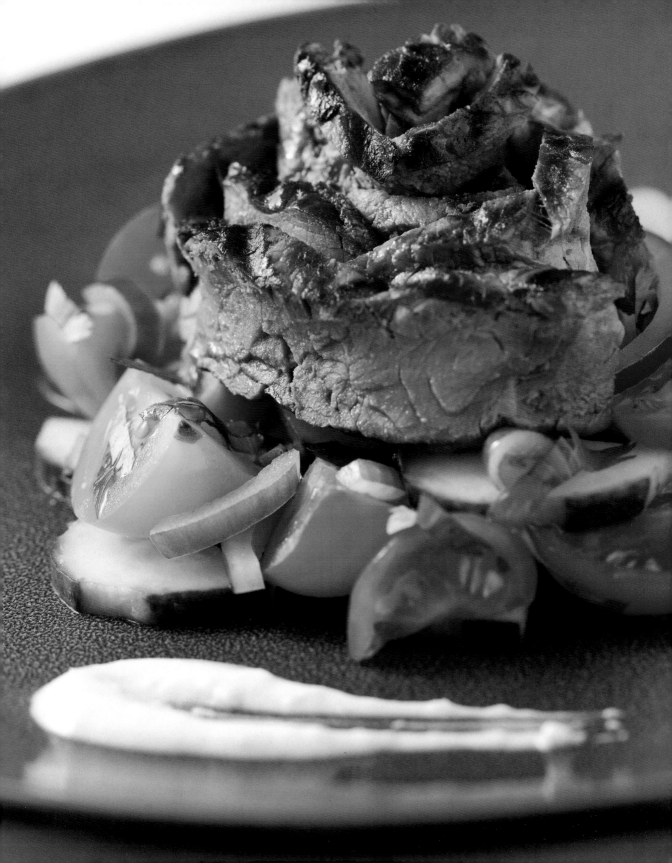

Steakhouse Salad
with Creamy Horseradish Sauce

serves 2–3

Salad Ingredients:

2 (6-ounce) beef tenderloin steaks, trimmed (about ¾–1-inch thick)

1 teaspoon extra-virgin olive oil

Salt and pepper to taste

1 package sweet butter lettuce blend (optional)

1 cup cherry tomatoes, halved

¼ cup red onion, thinly sliced

½ cup cucumber, thinly sliced

¼ cup freshly chopped basil or mint (optional)

Dressing Ingredients:

¾ cup Greek yogurt

¼ cup chopped red onion

2 teaspoons chopped fresh chives

2½ teaspoons prepared horseradish

½ teaspoon fresh lemon juice

¼ teaspoon freshly ground black pepper

Directions:

1. Lightly coat steaks with extra-virgin olive oil on both sides, and add salt and pepper. Place on grill rack and grill 5 minutes on each side or until desired temperature. Let stand 10 minutes before slicing.

2. While steak rests, divide lettuce, tomato, red onion, cucumber, and basil on 2 or 3 plates. For the dressing, combine all ingredients and drizzle evenly over the salad.

3. Top each salad with steak slices.

Mayo-Free Tuna Salad

serves 1

Ingredients:

1 egg
1 can chunk-light tuna packed in water
   (strain as much water out of can as
   possible)
1 tablespoon extra-virgin olive oil
1 tablespoon mustard
Handful of parsley, chopped
2 tablespoons red onion, diced
1 celery stalk (with leaves), chopped
4 cherry tomatoes, cut in half
½ avocado, diced
1 tablespoon sweet pickle relish (optional)
1 cup romaine lettuce, chopped (optional)

Directions:

1. Boil the egg first (this takes the longest).

2. As the egg is boiling, mix the can of tuna with all other ingredients except the romaine lettuce.

3. After the egg is done boiling (around 10–12 minutes), dice and mix into the salad.

4. Serve on a bed of romaine lettuce or enjoy by itself.

Pumpkin Chili

serves 4

Ingredients:

2 cups yellow onion, chopped
½ cup green onion, chopped
1 cup bell pepper, chopped
8 cloves garlic, chopped
1½ pounds ground turkey (omit for vegan
   option)
30 ounces jarred tomatoes
1 cup pinto beans, rinsed
1 cup kidney beans, rinsed
2 cups pumpkin puree
1 cup chicken broth (choose vegetable
   broth for vegan option)
1 tablespoon honey
Your favorite seasonings
1 tablespoon extra-virgin olive oil
1 avocado, sliced, and Greek yogurt for
   garnish (optional)

Directions:

1. In a large pot, sauté the onions, bell pepper, and garlic in extra-virgin olive oil.

2. Add the ground turkey, breaking it up into small chunks as it cooks for about 5 minutes.

3. Add the rest of the ingredients (except garnishes) and bring to a simmer; simmer uncovered for 15 minutes

4. Add more broth for thinner consistency.

5. Top with sliced avocado and dollop of Greek yogurt (optional).

Vegan Quinoa Fajita Bowl

serves 4

Ingredients:

1 tablespoon olive oil

1 red or yellow onion, sliced

1 each red, green, and yellow bell pepper, seeds removed and sliced

½ cup mushrooms, wiped clean and sliced

½ cup water

1 packet of fajita or taco seasoning (preferably a low-sodium brand)

Juice from 1 lime + more to squeeze over bowls

¼ cup chopped fresh cilantro

2 cups cooked quinoa (white or red)

1 can black beans, heated

2 large tomatoes, diced

2 cups Romaine lettuce, chopped

2 avocados, sliced

Directions:

1. Heat a large skillet over medium-high heat, add the olive oil, onions, and peppers; cook for 5 minutes or until tender.

2. Add the mushrooms, water, and fajita seasoning and thoroughly combine.

3. Add the fresh lime juice and cilantro, and cook until the mushrooms are tender. Remove from heat and set aside.

4. To assemble the fajita bowls, layer bowls with quinoa, black beans, fajita vegetables, tomatoes, lettuce, and avocado slices. Squeeze fresh lime juice over the bowls and serve.

5. Garnish with dollop of Greek yogurt and shredded cheese for non-vegan option.

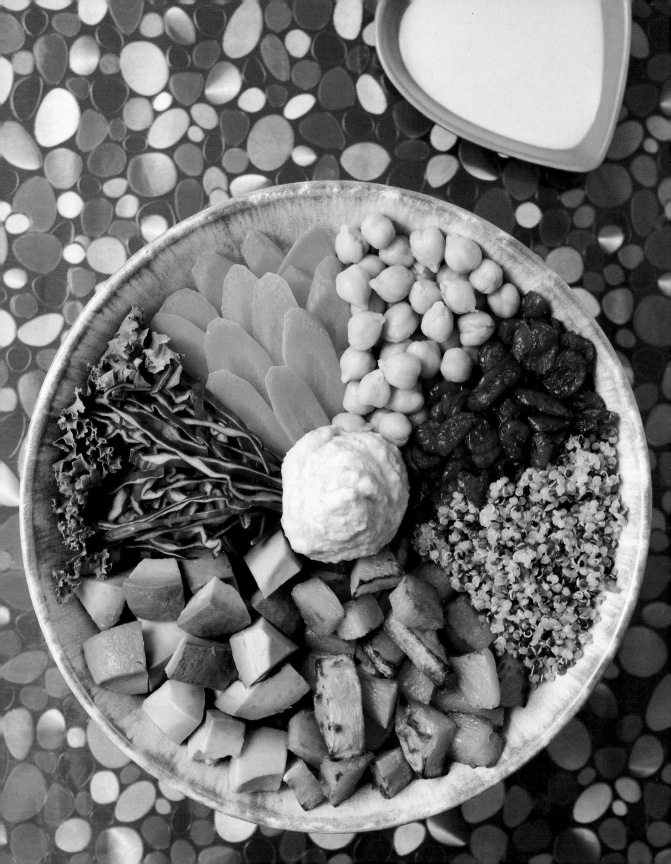

Deluxe Vegan Protein Bowl with Tahini Dressing

serves 1–2

Ingredients for bowl:

½ cup cubed butternut squash (optional)

1 tablespoon extra-virgin olive oil (for butternut squash)

Black pepper and garlic powder (for butternut squash)

1 cup curly kale or arugula

½ cup cooked red or white quinoa

2 tablespoons dried currants or cranberries (optional)

½ medium carrot, shredded

Handful shredded purple cabbage

¼ cup chickpeas

½ avocado, sliced

2 tablespoons hummus

Ingredients for Tahini Dressing:

¼ cup tahini

Juice of 1 lemon

2 cloves garlic, minced

Salt and pepper to taste

1 teaspoon real maple syrup (optional)

1–2 tablespoons water to thin

Directions:

1. Preheat oven to 400° F (if including butternut squash).

2. Toss cubed butternut squash in olive oil, black pepper, and garlic powder and place on a baking sheet.

3. Roast butternut squash for 25–30 minutes or until tender.

4. Meanwhile, place the kale or arugula at the bottom of your bowl; layer the quinoa on top and sprinkle with currants or cranberries (optional).

5. Arrange the shredded carrot, cabbage, chickpeas, avocado, hummus, and roasted butternut squash in groups on top of the quinoa and greens.

6. Combine all dressing ingredients thoroughly and drizzle on top.

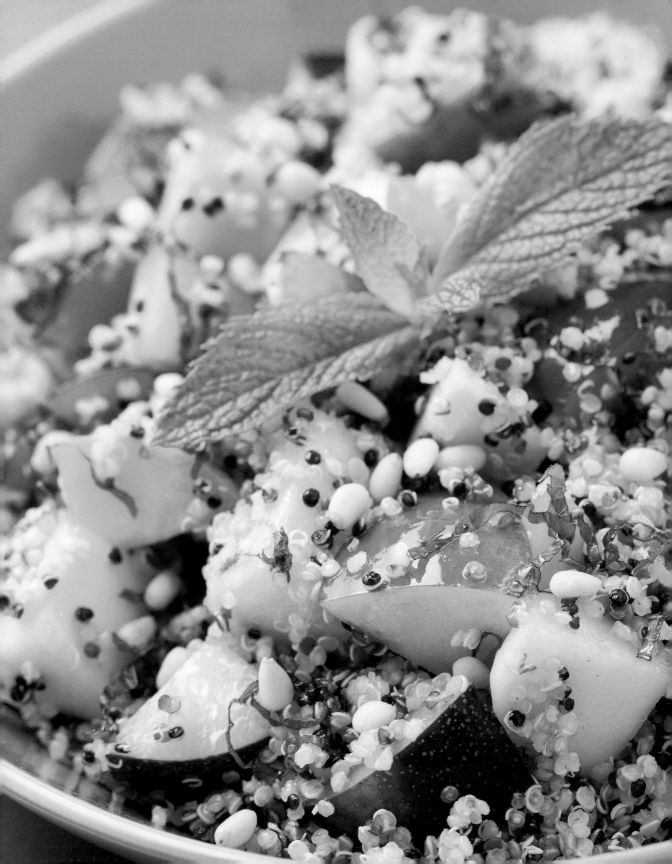

Quinoa Fruit Salad

serves 2–3

Ingredients:

2 cups cooked quinoa (red or white or a combination of both)
1 mango, peeled and diced
2 plums, chopped
1 cup strawberries, sliced
½ cup blueberries
2 tablespoons pine nuts
6 mint leaves, finely chopped

Dressing Ingredients:

¼ cup extra-virgin olive oil
¼ cup apple cider vinegar
Zest of 1 lemon
3 tablespoons freshly squeezed lemon juice
1 teaspoon honey or agave

Directions:

1. Whisk together all dressing ingredients and set aside.

2. In a large bowl, combine all salad ingredients and then toss in dressing.

3. Optional: add grilled chicken for added protein.

Bean Trio Salad

serves 3

Salad Ingredients:

1 can garbanzo beans
1 can kidney beans
Fresh green beans
¼ cup diced red onion
¼ cup diced green onion
¼ cup chopped parsley or cilantro

Dressing Ingredients:

2 tablespoons extra-virgin olive oil
1½ tablespoon apple cider vinegar
1 teaspoon minced garlic
Juice of 2 limes
1 teaspoon honey
1 teaspoon chopped ginger
Black pepper to taste

Directions:

1. Blanch your green beans by boiling in a pot of water for 1-2 minutes to desired tenderness, then immediately rinse in cold water to stop the cooking.

2. Combine all salad ingredients in a large bowl.

3. Whisk together all dressing ingredients and toss with the salad.

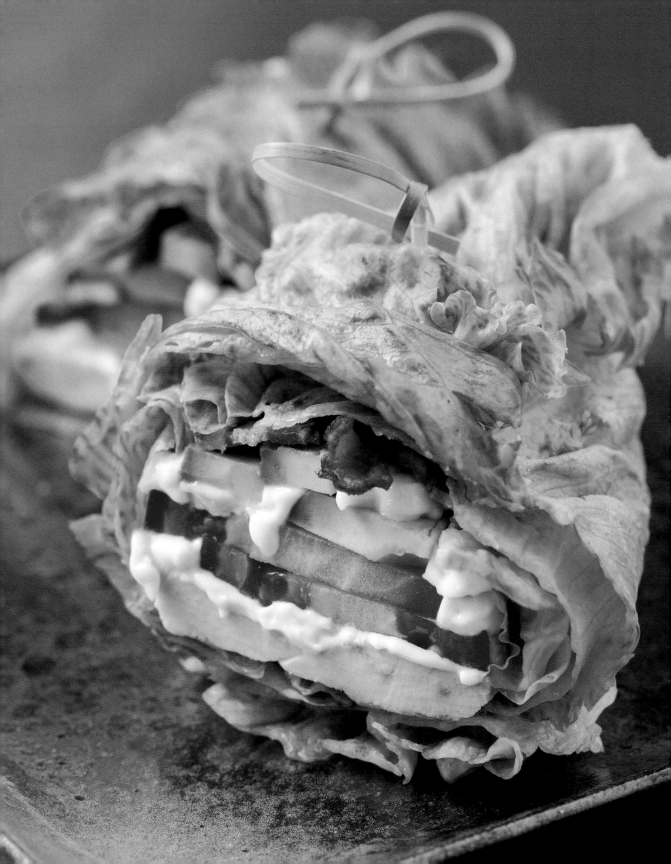

Turkey Bacon Avocado Lettuce Wrap

serves 2

Ingredients:

2 large iceberg lettuce leaves

1 cup boneless, skinless turkey breast, shredded or chopped

2 tablespoons avocado oil mayonnaise (sold in most major grocery stores)

4 slices nitrate-free bacon, cooked

1 avocado, sliced

1 Roma tomato, thinly sliced

Directions:

1. Lay out the lettuce leaves on a cutting board (one for each wrap).

2. Toss turkey with two tablespoons of avocado oil mayo, divide evenly in half and place on each lettuce leaf.

3. Layer two slices of bacon on top of the turkey in each wrap, followed by slices of avocado and then tomato.

4. Fold the bottom up, the sides in, and roll like a burrito. Slice in half and serve cold.

Teriyaki Tempeh Lettuce Cups

serves 2–3

Ingredients:

⅓ cup tamari

1 tablespoon real maple syrup

1 tablespoon rice vinegar

2 teaspoons garlic, minced (about 4 cloves)

1½ teaspoons sesame oil

¼ teaspoon ground ginger

8-ounce package tempeh

1 tablespoon coconut oil

1 onion, thinly sliced

1 medium carrot, thinly sliced

Salt and pepper, to taste

1 head butter lettuce

Green onions, thinly sliced, for topping

Directions:

1. In a medium bowl, add tamari, maple syrup, vinegar, garlic, sesame oil, and ginger. Whisk to combine.

2. Crumble the tempeh into small chunks and place in the mixture; stir to coat and set aside.

3. In a medium skillet or wok over medium-low heat, warm coconut oil. Add the onion and carrot and cook for 5–7 minutes or until softened. Season to taste.

4. Pour the tempeh mixture into the pan and cook for 5 minutes while stirring until the tempeh starts to brown.

5. Spoon the tempeh mixture into lettuce cups and top with sliced green onions.

Lentil & Hummus Lettuce Cups

serves 1

Ingredients:

½ cup cooked lentils
2 tablespoons hummus
2–3 lettuce leaves of your choice
¼ cup green onions, chopped
¼ tomatoes, diced

Directions:

1. Mix lentils with hummus.

2. Scoop into 2 or 3 lettuce cups.

3. Top with onions and tomato.

Blueberry Walnut Chicken Salad

serves 2–3

Ingredients:

2 boneless, skinless chicken breasts, cooked, cooled, and cut into small cubes
½ cup fresh blueberries
¼ cup diced celery
¼ cup diced red onion
3 tablespoons chopped walnuts
1 tablespoon fresh rosemary leaves, chopped
¼ teaspoon sea salt
½ teaspoon black pepper
½ cup avocado oil mayonnaise, or 2 tablespoons whole Greek yogurt mixed with 2 tablespoons crème fraîche

Directions:

1. Combine cooked chicken and remaining ingredients in a bowl and gently stir to combine.

2. Serve with butter lettuce wraps, over a bed of mixed greens, or in endive leaves.

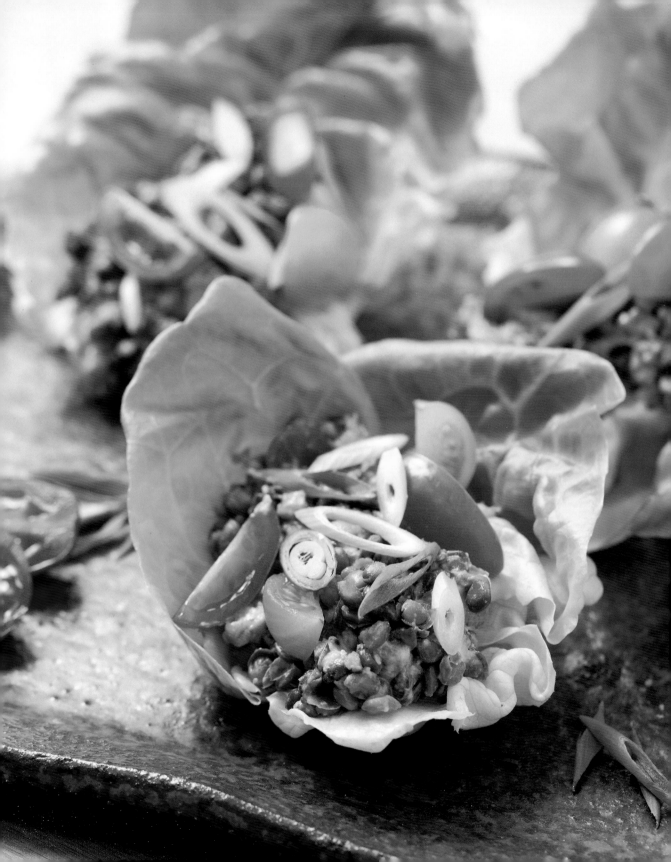

California Chicken Burrito Bowl

serves 1

Ingredients:

1 boneless, skinless chicken breast

2 cups romaine lettuce, chopped

½ cup black beans

½ cup salsa or pico de gallo

½ avocado, sliced

Handful sprouts

1 tablespoon Greek yogurt

1 tablespoon cilantro, chopped

Directions:

1. Grill or pan-cook chicken breast with favorite seasonings; chop and set aside.

2. Arrange the lettuce in a bowl and evenly distribute beans on top.

3. Pour salsa or pico de gallo over the beans.

4. Place chicken, avocado, sprouts, Greek yogurt, and cilantro on top of salad.

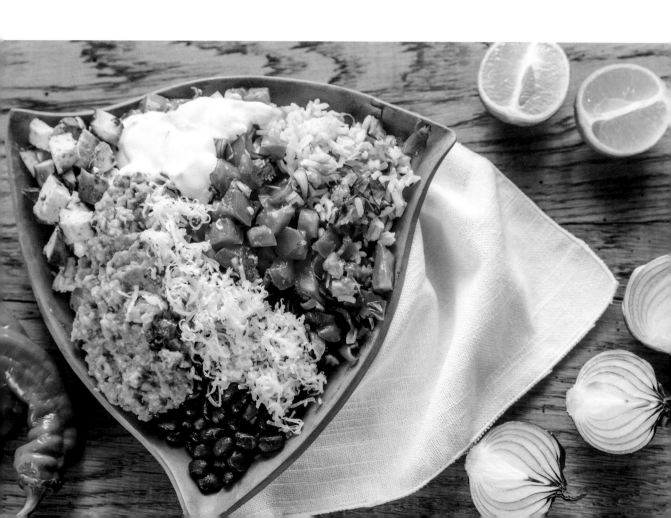

Mediterranean Quinoa Bowl

serves 1

Ingredients:

1 cup quinoa, cooked
½ cup cucumber, diced
½ avocado, sliced
Cherry tomatoes, halved
¼ cup feta cheese, crumbled (optional)
Olives to taste (optional)

Dressing Ingredients:

½ tablespoon extra-virgin olive oil
½ tablespoon balsamic vinegar
Freshly squeezed lemon to taste

Directions:

1. Place all salad ingredients in a bowl.

2. Whisk all dressing ingredients together and toss with salad.

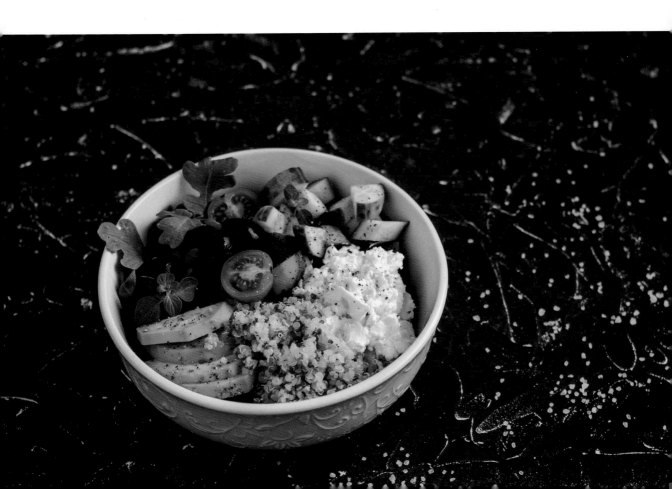

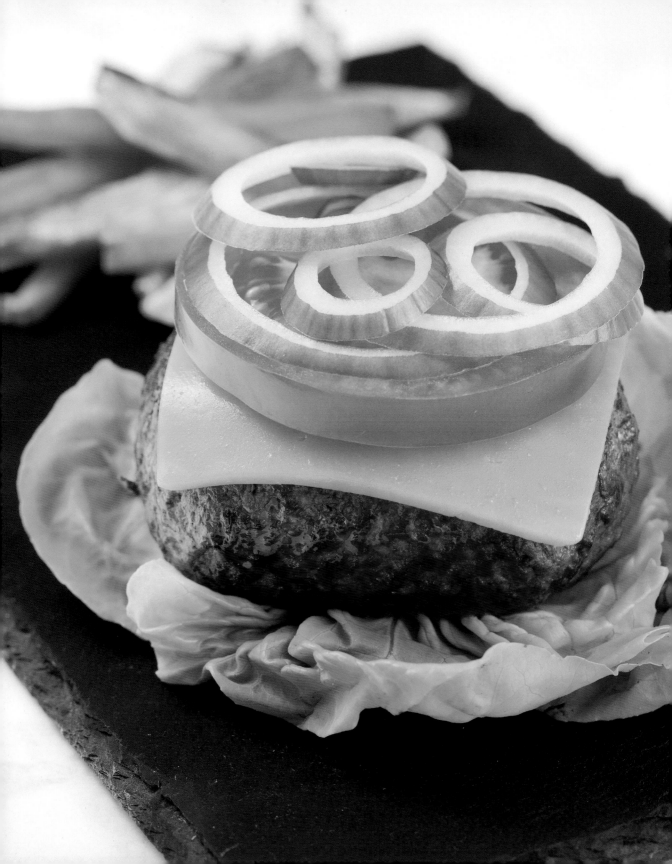

Burger and Fries

serves 2

Ingredients:

1 medium sweet potato
1 tablespoon extra-virgin olive oil
6 ounces ground beef
Black pepper to taste
Garlic powder to taste
Oregano to taste
2 slices favorite cheese (optional)
1 medium tomato
2 slices raw onion
Handful favorite lettuce leaves
1 small avocado

Directions:

1. Preheat oven to 350° F.

2. Thinly slice the sweet potato into round disks and evenly toss with one tablespoon of extra-virgin olive oil, black pepper, and garlic powder.

3. Place the sweet potatoes on a baking sheet and bake for 20 minutes or until tender.

4. While the sweet potatoes are baking, divide ground beef into two patties and season with ground pepper, garlic, and oregano. Grill or pan-cook over medium heat until cooked through to your liking.

5. If you are using cheese, top each burger with one slice of your favorite cheese while there is 1 minute left of cooking.

6. Plate the burger with sliced tomato, onion, avocado, lettuce leaves, and sweet potato fries.

7. Serve with mustard or a small dollop of ketchup.

The "No Lettuce" Shrimp Salad

serves 3-4

Ingredients:

2 cups frozen peas

12 ounces bay shrimp (no need to remove shells or devein as these come precooked)

½ cup green onions, thinly sliced

1 tablespoon tarragon, chopped

1 tablespoon flat leaf parsley, chopped

2 teaspoons fresh mint, chopped

1 tablespoon fresh lemon juice

½ cup nitrate-free bacon, cooked and chopped (optional)

1 bunch radish, sliced thin

Horseradish Crème Fraîche Ingredients:

½ cup crème fraîche

½ cup plain Greek yogurt

4 tablespoons fresh horseradish, grated

1 teaspoon lemon zest

1 tablespoon lemon juice

Salt and pepper to taste

Directions:

1. Bring 3-4 cups of water to a boil and place peas in the pot; boil for 2-3 minutes and immediately return cooked peas to an ice bath to chill and prevent them from cooking further.

2. In a medium bowl, combine peas, bay shrimp, green onions, tarragon, parsley, mint, and lemon juice; set aside in the refrigerator.

3. Meanwhile, in a medium pan over medium heat cook bacon until crispy; remove from heat and drain on paper towel. Prepare the Horseradish Crème Fraîche by combining all ingredients in a bowl and set aside.

4. To serve, scoop the shrimp and pea mixture onto salad plates and smear a generous dollop of Horseradish Crème Fraîche next to the salad as a dip garnish. Arrange bacon pieces and sliced radishes on top.

Avocado-Feta Chickpea Salad

serves 2–3

Salad Ingredients:

4 cups shredded romaine or butter lettuce
1 can chickpeas, rinsed and drained
1 cup cherry tomatoes, halved
½ cup feta cheese, crumbled
2 avocados, sliced
½ cup diced red onion
Salt and black pepper, to taste

Dressing:

2 tablespoons olive oil
1 tablespoon balsamic vinegar

Directions:

1. In a medium bowl, combine salad ingredients. Set aside.

2. Whisk the dressing ingredients together and toss with salad; season with salt and pepper to taste.

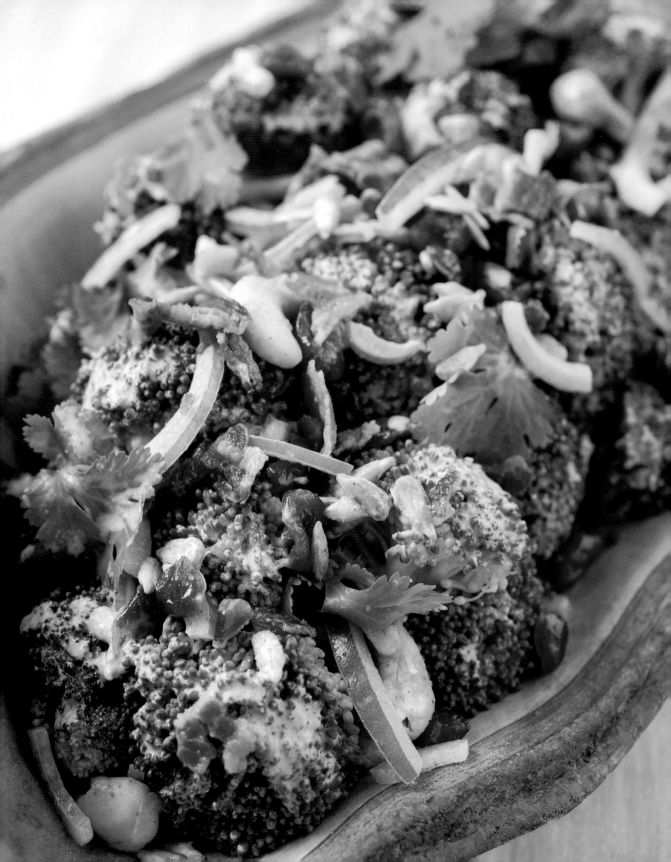

Cashew Curry Broccoli Salad

serves 3

Dressing Ingredients:

½ cup tahini
5 tablespoons water (you may need less or more to reach desired consistency of dressing)
4 teaspoons yellow curry powder
2 teaspoons real maple syrup or honey
½ teaspoon salt
Pinch of pepper

Salad Ingredients:

4 cups broccoli florets, cut into bite-sized pieces
¼ cup red onion, diced
½ cup cilantro, chopped
2 pieces nitrate-free bacon, cooked and chopped (optional)
¼ cup dried currants or cranberries, roughly chopped
2 tablespoons sunflower seeds
2 tablespoons raw cashews, roughly chopped

Directions:

1. Combine all dressing ingredients until smooth; set aside.

2. In a large bowl combine the broccoli, red onion, cilantro, bacon (if using), and currants or cranberries.

3. Combine the broccoli salad with dressing until evenly mixed. Cover and let sit for at least an hour.

4. Just before serving, mix in the sunflower seeds and cashews.

Turkey or Chicken Lettuce Cups

serves 1

Ingredients:

½ pound boneless, skinless turkey or chicken breast
1 teaspoon extra-virgin olive oil
Your favorite seasonings
2–3 lettuce leaves of choice
Mustard to taste
1 tablespoon onion, finely chopped
¼ cup tomatoes, diced
½ avocado, diced

Directions:

1. Pan-cook or grill the turkey or chicken with extra-virgin olive oil and your favorite seasonings. After cooking through, let cool and then chop into small pieces.

2. Place the turkey or chicken in two or three lettuce cups.

3. Top with mustard, onions, tomatoes, and avocado.

Watermelon Caprese Salad

serves 2

Ingredients:

1 cup arugula
2 teaspoons extra-virgin olive oil
2 teaspoons balsamic vinegar
½ cup watermelon, chopped into cubes
½ cup fresh mozzarella, chopped
½ cup cherry tomatoes, halved
¼ cup red onion, sliced
Salt to taste

Directions:

1. Evenly toss the arugula with olive oil and balsamic vinegar.

2. Arrange the watermelon, cheese, cherry tomatoes, and red onion on top of the arugula and sprinkle with salt.

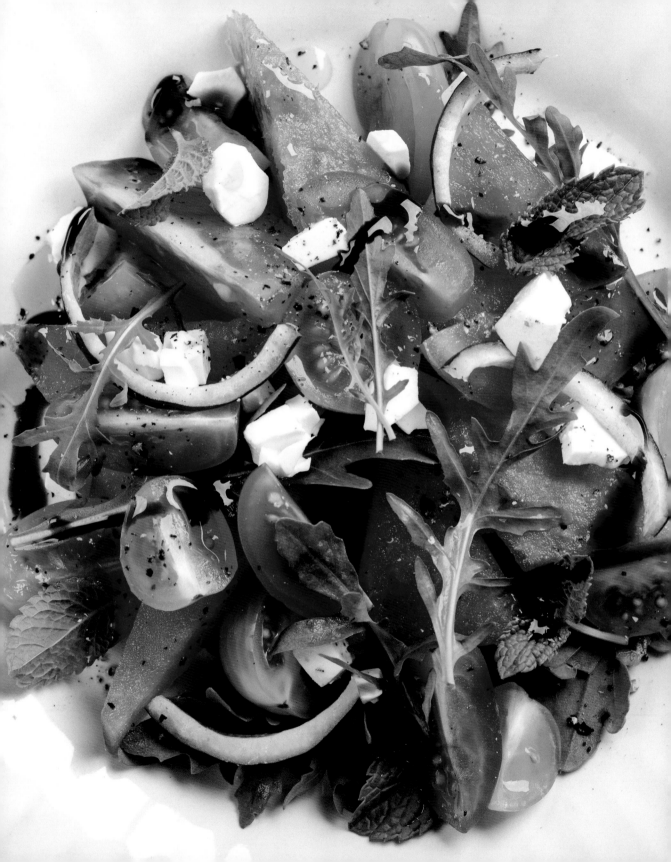

Kale-Pomegranate Salad

serves 2–3

Ingredients:

4 cups chopped kale

½ cup cooked quinoa

1 avocado, diced

½ cup pomegranate arils

½ cup chopped pecans

¼ cup crumbled goat cheese (omit for
   Vegan option)

Salad Dressing:

¼ cup extra-virgin olive oil

¼ cup apple cider vinegar

3 tablespoons freshly squeezed lemon juice

Zest of 1 lemon

1 teaspoon honey or agave

Directions:

1. To make the vinaigrette, whisk all dressing ingredients together and set aside.

2. To assemble the salad, place kale in a large bowl; top with quinoa, avocado, pomegranate arils, pecans, and goat cheese (if using).

3. Pour the dressing on top of the salad and gently toss to combine.

Avocado-Hummus Deviled Egg Salad

serves 2

Ingredients:

5 hard-boiled eggs, peeled

1 ripe avocado, mashed

3 tablespoons hummus

1–2 tablespoons fresh squeezed lemon juice

½ teaspoon sea salt

2 strips of nitrate-free bacon, cooked and chopped
   (optional)

2–3 tablespoons chives or green onions, chopped

2–3 dashes smoked paprika

Your favorite vegetables, sliced

Directions:

1. Chop your eggs and place in a large bowl.

2. Add mashed avocado and hummus to the bowl and combine with eggs.

3. Add the lemon juice, salt, bacon, and green onions and mix well; sprinkle with smoked paprika.

4. Serve with fresh vegetables of choice for dipping.

Lunch Snack Pack

serves 1

Ingredients:

1 small container Greek yogurt
8 strawberries
¼ cup raw cashews
½ cup hummus
Raw broccoli florets and/or celery sticks
1 hard-boiled egg

Directions:

1. Package all ingredients in a portable container and refrigerate.

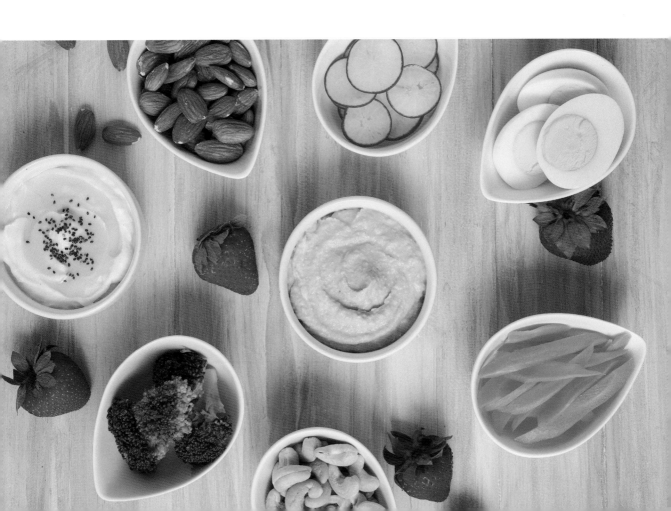

Egg Rolls in a Bowl

serves 4

Ingredients:

1 tablespoon coconut oil
1 small head of cabbage, shredded or thinly sliced
2 large carrots, shredded or thinly sliced
1 tablespoon sesame oil
2 garlic cloves, minced
1 tablespoon sesame seeds
1 teaspoon grated ginger
4 green onions, diced
1½ pounds of boneless, skinless chicken breast or shrimp
1 tablespoon extra-virgin olive oil

Directions:

1. Melt the coconut oil over medium heat and add the cabbage and carrots.

2. Sauté until soft. While sautéing, add 1–2 tablespoons of water to create steam in order to soften without drying out.

3. Add the sesame oil and sauté until you have reached desired tenderness.

4. Add the garlic, sesame seeds, and grated ginger and cook until fragrant.

5. In a separate pan, cook chicken or shrimp using extra-virgin olive oil. Once chicken or shrimp is cooked through, toss with the cabbage mixture and top with green onions.

Chinese Chicken Salad

serves 4–5

Ingredients:

¼ cup tamari

¼ cup white wine vinegar

3 tablespoons ginger, minced

3 tablespoons extra-virgin olive oil

2 tablespoons hoisin sauce

1 tablespoon toasted sesame oil

5 green onions, chopped (include all green and white parts)

1 large head Napa cabbage, chopped into thin strips

2 cups shredded carrots

½ cup cilantro, chopped

4 tablespoons sesame seeds (black or white or a combination of both)

½ cup cashews (optional)

1 rotisserie chicken, torn into shreds

Directions:

1. In a bowl, whisk tamari, vinegar, minced ginger, olive oil, hoisin sauce, toasted sesame oil, and chopped green onions until evenly incorporated. Set aside.

2. Put chopped cabbage, shredded carrots, cilantro, sesame seeds, cashews, and shredded chicken in a large bowl. Use half of the dressing and evenly toss it throughout the salad (this amount may be enough for you or you may want to add more). Keep adding more dressing and continue to toss until you reach desired taste.

3. This salad holds up well in the refrigerator so feel free to make a large batch.

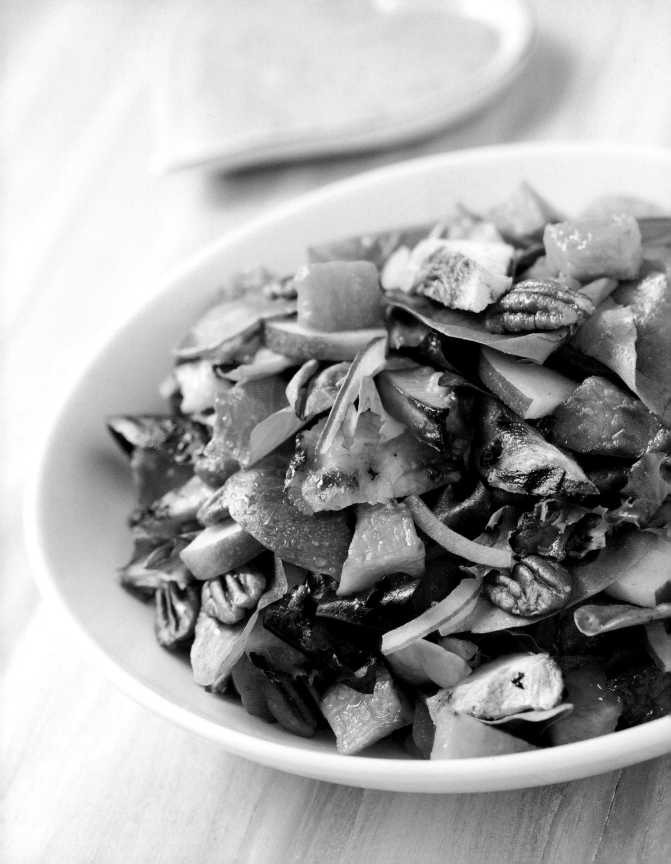

Maple Pecan Chicken Salad with Roasted Butternut Squash

serves 3–4

Ingredients for Chicken:

1 pound chicken tenderloins (omit chicken for vegan option)

1 tablespoon extra-virgin olive oil

Salt, pepper, and onion powder, to taste

1 teaspoon lemon juice

Ingredients for Salad:

3 cups butternut squash, cut into 1-inch cubes

1 tablespoon extra-virgin olive oil

3 cups of your favorite salad greens

1 large apple, sliced thin

1 cup raw pecan halves, roughly chopped

½ cup red onion, diced

Ingredients for Maple Dressing:

1 cup full-fat coconut milk

3 teaspoons apple cider vinegar

1 teaspoon fresh lemon juice

2 teaspoons pure maple syrup

2 teaspoons brown mustard

Dash of salt

Directions:

1. Combine all dressing ingredients in a blender and set aside in the refrigerator.

2. Preheat your oven to 425° F. Toss the cubed butternut squash in one tablespoon extra-virgin olive oil and lightly sprinkle with salt and pepper to taste. Place on a baking sheet and roast for 30 minutes or until tender.

3. Heat a pan over medium-high heat.

4. Mix one tablespoon extra-virgin olive oil and lemon juice; coat the chicken pieces in the mixture, and sprinkle with salt, pepper, and onion powder.

5. Pan-cook the tenders for 3 minutes on each side or until cooked through; remove from heat and set aside.

6. Chop the chicken into bite-sized pieces and arrange the salad starting with greens, sliced apples, roasted butternut squash, chicken, pecans, and onions. Serve with dressing drizzled over the top.

Black-Eyed Pea and Arugula Salad

serves 2

Ingredients:

1 cup grape tomatoes, halved

2½ tablespoons avocado oil mayonnaise

2 tablespoons red wine vinegar

Ground pepper to taste

1 (15-oz.) can unsalted black-eyed peas, rinsed and drained

Handful of dried currants or cranberries (optional)

2 cups arugula

Directions:

1. Combine all ingredients (except arugula) in a large bowl, stirring to coat. Add arugula and toss gently to combine.

Spinach and Fruit Salad Jar

serves 1

Salad Ingredients:

1 cup fresh spinach

½ peach, sliced

¼ cup blueberries

¼ crumbled goat cheese (optional)

¼ cup walnuts, chopped

Dressing Ingredients:

1 teaspoon extra-virgin olive oil

1 lemon, juiced

Black pepper to taste

Directions:

1. Layer all salad ingredients in a jar.

2. Combine all dressing ingredients and pour over salad; add lid and shake to toss salad.

3. To preserve the salad, pour dressing in bottom of jar and then layer salad ingredients from bottom to top: walnuts, blueberries, peach, goat cheese, and spinach on top. Wait until lunch time to shake.

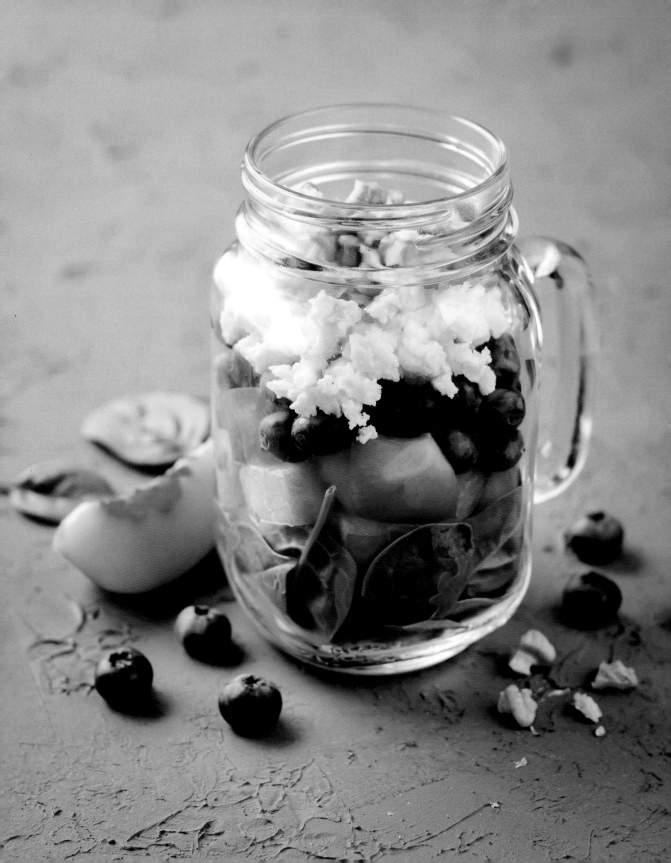

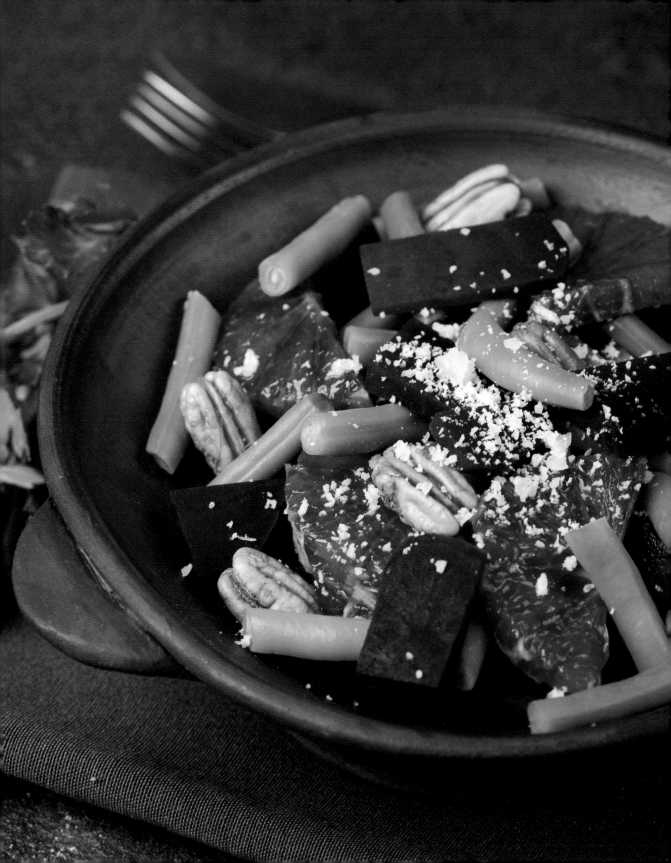

Beets, Beans & Citrus Salad

serves 4

Ingredients:

1 pound beets, peeled and cut into wedges

1 tablespoon extra-virgin olive oil

1 large orange or blood orange

Handful of pecans

1 cup unsalted cannellini beans

1 tablespoon fresh cilantro, chopped

1 tablespoon sherry vinegar

¼ teaspoon black pepper

Grated Parmesan (optional)

Directions:

1. Preheat oven to 375° F.

2. Toss beets in extra-virgin olive, wrap in aluminum foil, and place on a baking sheet and roast until tender (around 55–60 minutes). This can be done ahead of time (alternatively, wrap beets in parchment paper and microwave for 12 minutes).

3. In the meantime, peel the orange and cut into segments.

4. Combine beets, orange segments, pecans, and cannellini beans in a large bowl and sprinkle with cilantro, vinegar, and pepper. Top with Parmesan if desired.

5. Plate to serve.

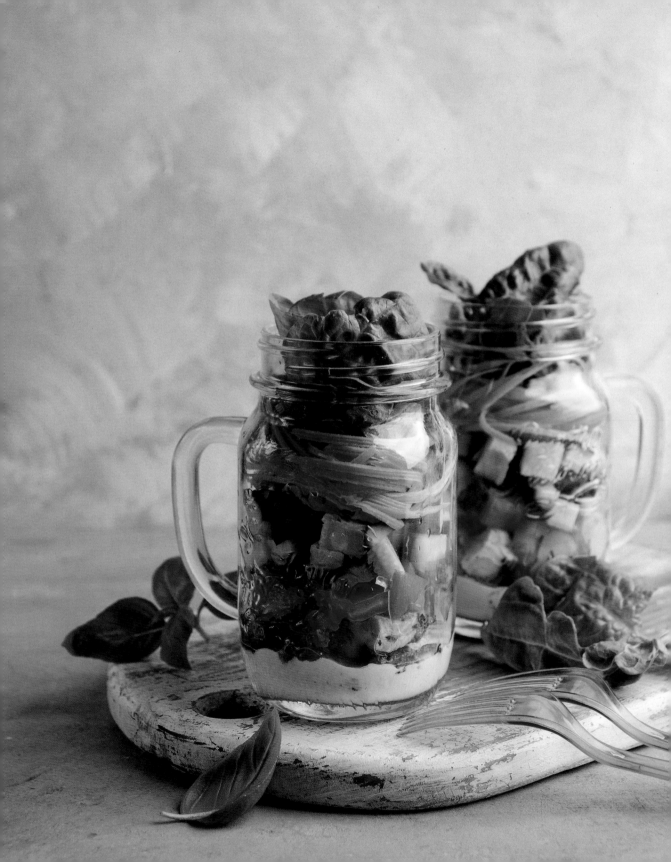

Salad Jar to Go

serves 1

Ingredients:

1-2 cups lettuce, chopped
¼ cup cucumber, diced
¼ cup tomato, chopped
1 tablespoon onion, diced

½ carrot, shredded
Your favorite protein of choice (optional)
Your favorite salad dressing

Directions:

1. Pour your salad dressing into the bottom of the jar (or any container that has a lid)

2. Layer the rest of the salad ingredients on top of the dressing, ending with the lettuce at the very top.

3. When ready to serve, shake the jar or container to toss dressing throughout salad.

Spaghetti Squash Salad

serves 3-4

Salad Ingredients:

1 medium spaghetti squash (4 cups of flesh)
1 tablespoon extra-virgin olive oil
Salt and pepper to taste
1 small red onion, diced
1 red pepper, diced
1 yellow pepper, diced
¼ cup fresh basil, thinly sliced
½ cup sun-dried tomatoes

Dressing Ingredients:

¼ cup extra-virgin olive oil
¼ cup apple cider vinegar
2-3 cloves garlic, crushed
1 teaspoon dried oregano
½ teaspoon salt
½ teaspoon mustard powder (optional)

Directions:

1. Preheat oven to 400° F.

2. Slice squash in half, lengthwise, and remove strings and seeds.

3. Lightly coat with extra-virgin olive oil and season with salt and pepper.

4. Place face down on a foil–lined baking sheet and bake at 400° F for 35–45 minutes or until tender.

5. After the squash is cool, use a fork to shred into "noodles."

6. Combine noodles with all other salad ingredients.

7. Whisk all dressing ingredients together.

8. Pour over salad, then toss and serve.

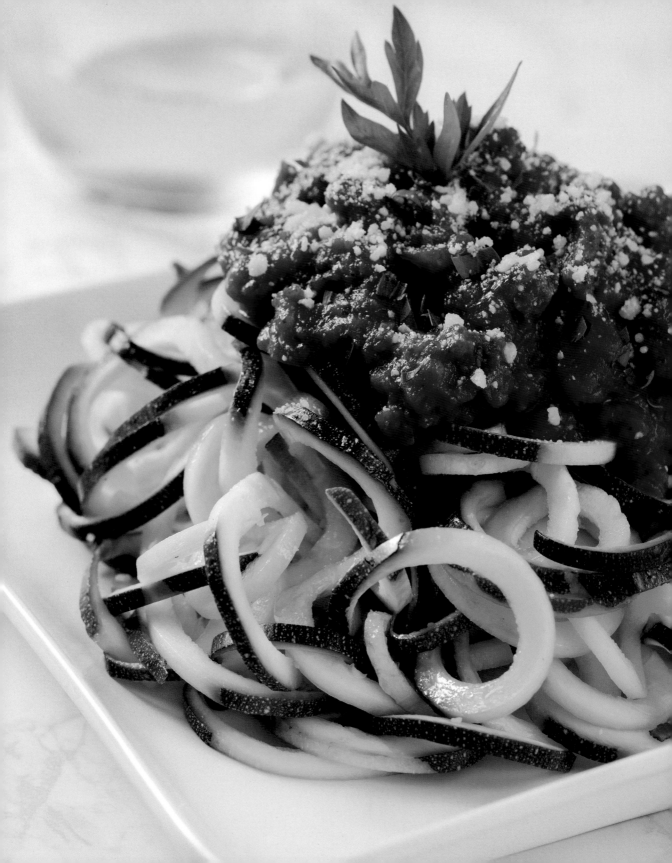

Easy Turkey Ragu with Zoodles

serves 4

Ingredients:

1 tablespoon extra-virgin olive oil

2 pounds ground turkey (you can use beef or chicken if you prefer)

2 cups store-bought tomato-based pasta sauce (look for ingredient labels which have natural and minimal ingredients such as tomatoes, tomato paste, onion, garlic, and extra-virgin olive oil)

4 tablespoons freshly chopped parsley

4 medium zucchini (one per serving)

Grated Parmesan, optional

Directions:

1. Using extra-virgin olive oil, cook the meat in a pan over medium-high heat for 8 minutes until browned on all sides.

2. Add pasta sauce and fresh parsley and continue to cook on medium heat for 3–5 minutes. Transfer to a bowl when done.

3. While your meat sauce is cooking, use a spiralizer to create your zucchini noodles. If you do not have a spiralizer, you can use a julienne peeler to peel the zucchini all around until you get to the soft center.

4. Using the same meat saucepan, cook the zoodles over medium heat for 3–5 minutes until you reach desired tenderness. Add the meat sauce back into the pan and combine with the zoodles. Top with grated Parmesan cheese (optional).

Chapter 20:
The Whole Food Pregnancy Dinner Recipes

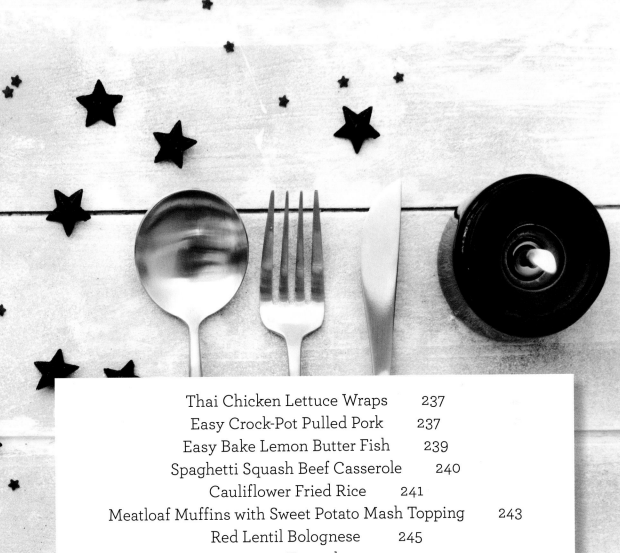

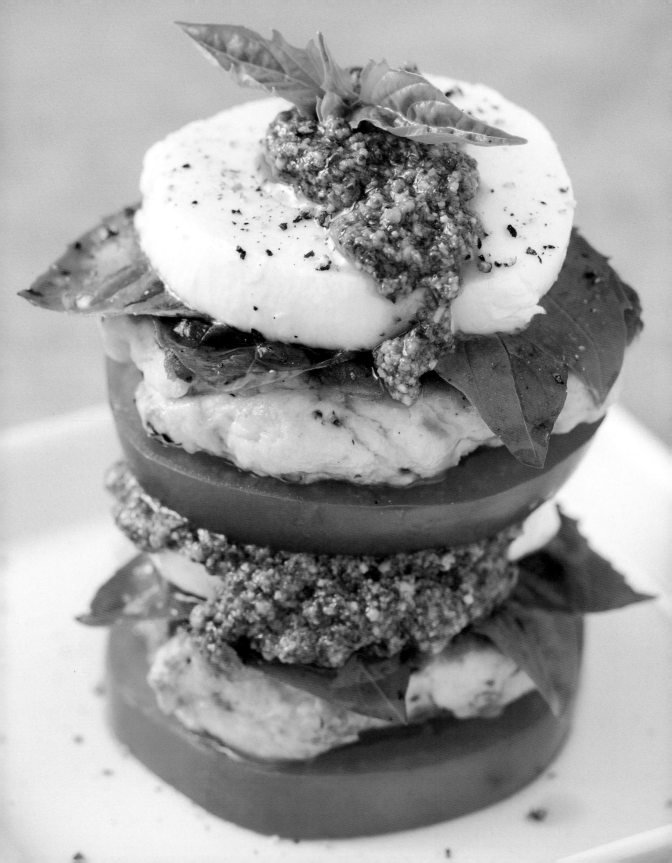

Caprese Turkey Burgers

serves 2

Ingredients:

6 ounces lean ground turkey

¼ teaspoon garlic powder

1 tablespoon almond flour

Pepper, to taste

2 slices mozzarella cheese

2 tablespoons pesto sauce (store bought, or combine extra-virgin olive oil, fresh basil, pine nuts, and garlic in a food processor)

2 (½-inch thick) slices tomato

Handful of basil

Directions:

1. Combine ground turkey, garlic powder, almond flour, and pepper.

2. Form two patties.

3. Place patties on an aluminum foil-lined baking sheet. Broil on high for 3 minutes on each side.

4. Add 1 slice of mozzarella on each burger at the last minute to melt.

5. Place burgers on a plate, top each one with 1 tablespoon of pesto sauce, one tomato slice, and a handful of basil.

Balsamic Crock-Pot Chicken

serves 4–6

Ingredients:

1 teaspoon garlic powder

1 teaspoon dried basil

½ teaspoon pepper

2 teaspoons dried minced onion

8 boneless, skinless chicken thighs

1 tablespoon extra-virgin olive oil

4 garlic cloves, minced

½ cup balsamic vinegar

Sprinkle of fresh chopped parsley or cilantro

Directions:

1. Combine the first 4 dry spices in a small bowl and season both sides of the chicken; set aside.

2. Pour olive oil and garlic on the bottom of the Crock-Pot and place chicken on top.

3. Pour balsamic vinegar over the chicken, cover, and cook on high for 4 hours.

4. Sprinkle with fresh parsley or cilantro on top to serve.

Cheesy Chicken and Broccoli Casserole

serves 3-4

Ingredients:

Extra-virgin olive oil, for greasing

1 cup uncooked quinoa

3 tablespoons almond meal

Your favorite seasonings

2 cups chicken broth (low sodium)

1 cup unsweetened almond milk

1 pound boneless skinless chicken breasts, chopped into bite-size chunks

4 cups fresh broccoli florets

1½ cups of your favorite shredded cheese

Directions:

1. Preheat oven to 400° F; use extra-virgin olive oil to grease a 13 x 9-inch baking dish.

2. Add quinoa, almond meal, seasonings, chicken broth, and milk to the dish and whisk together.

3. Add the chicken and broccoli, stirring to distribute into an even layer.

4. Cover with foil and bake for 20 minutes.

5. Add the cheese to the casserole and stir well to combine; return to the oven for 20 minutes, uncovered.

6. Remove from the oven again to stir, and cook another 20 minutes until chicken is cooked through and quinoa is soft (total baking time is 1 hour).

Quinoa Burger

makes 4–6 burgers

Ingredients:

1 cup Portobello mushroom, diced

1 cup quinoa, cooked

½ red bell pepper, diced

½ yellow onion, diced

½ cup parsley, minced

2 cloves garlic, minced

¼ cup extra-virgin olive oil (+ more for the pan)

2 tablespoons flaxseed meal

2 teaspoons tamari

Salt and pepper to taste

Directions:

1. Place all ingredients in a food processor or blender and pulse until desired consistency.
2. Form the mixture into 4–6 patties.
3. Heat 1-2 tablespoons extra-virgin olive oil over medium heat.
4. Place patties in pan and sear for about 5 minutes on each side.
5. Serve with lettuce, tomato, onion, avocado, and mustard.

Fish and Chips

serves 2

Ingredients:

1 medium sweet potato (if you prefer a regular white potato, that is fine too)

1 tablespoon extra-virgin olive oil

1 teaspoon garlic powder

1 cup almond flour

2 eggs

1 teaspoon salt

½ cup coconut milk

1 pound wild-caught cod

Avocado oil for frying

Directions:

1. Preheat oven to 375° F.
2. Slice sweet potato into strips and toss with extra-virgin olive oil and garlic powder. Place on a baking sheet and roast for 20 minutes or until tender.
3. Meanwhile, combine almond flour, eggs, salt, and coconut milk in a food processor or blender until well mixed.
4. Cut cod into thin strips.
5. Pour avocado oil to depth of ½ inch in a large skillet and heat it over medium-high heat just until it's nearly at the smoking point.
6. Coat the cod strips in your prepared batter and fry for 2 minutes per side or until golden brown. Remove cooked fillets from pan and place them on paper towels to drain.

Baked Seven Layer Dip Casserole

serves 3-4

Ingredients:

1 pound boneless, skinless chicken breast
½ medium onion, diced
1 tablespoon extra-virgin olive oil
1 can black beans
1 cup green tomatillo sauce
½ cup grated cheese of choice
1 tomato, diced
½ cup green onions, chopped
Greek yogurt, avocado, and cilantro for garnish

Directions:

1. Preheat oven to 350° F.

2. Cube the raw chicken and pan-cook over medium heat with chopped onions and extra-virgin olive oil until chicken is almost cooked through.

3. In a 9 x 13-inch baking dish, layer black beans over the bottom, the cooked chicken and onions, then the green tomatillo sauce, and bake for 12 minutes.

4. With 3 minutes of baking time left, remove from oven and top with grated cheese, diced tomatoes, and green onions. Return to oven for 3 minutes or until cheese is melted.

5. Serve warm, topped with Greek yogurt, avocado, and cilantro.

Honey Mustard Salmon

serves 3-4

Ingredients:

1½ pounds salmon, skin removed, cut into 4 pieces
2 tablespoons whole grain mustard (you can use regular mustard if you like)
2 tablespoons honey
1 clove garlic, minced
Juice of ½ a lemon

Directions:

1. Preheat oven to 400° F.

2. Place salmon pieces on a sheet pan lined with parchment paper; bake for 10 minutes.

3. Meanwhile, in a small bowl, combine mustard, honey, garlic, and lemon juice.

4. After first 10 minutes of cooking, brush salmon with mixture and return to the oven for 5 minutes or until salmon is just cooked through.

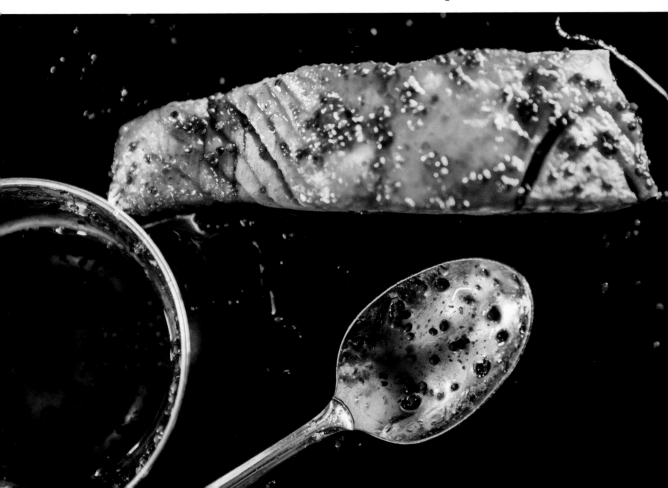

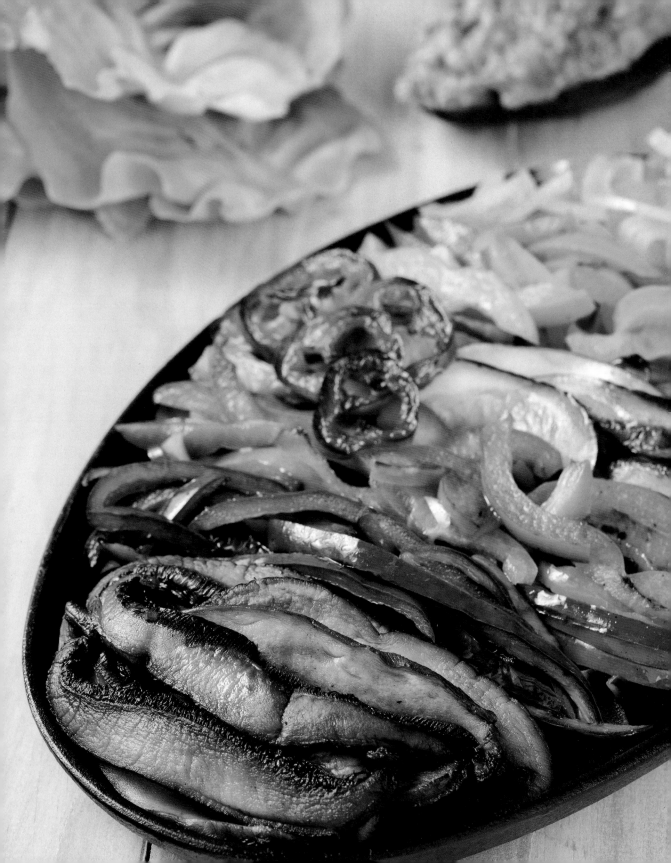

Mushroom, Zucchini, and Pepper Lettuce Wrap Fajitas

serves 3-4

Ingredients:

1 tablespoon extra-virgin olive oil
1 yellow onion, sliced
1 poblano pepper, seeds removed and thinly sliced
2 bell peppers, seeds removed and thinly sliced
1 jalapeño, seeds removed and thinly sliced (optional)
1 zucchini, thinly sliced
2 large Portobello mushrooms, thinly sliced
2 ripe avocados
Juice of 1 lime
Salt, cumin, and garlic powder to taste
1 head of butter lettuce
Diced red onion, salsa, pico de gallo, and cilantro, for garnish (optional)

Directions:

1. Heat a large skillet over medium-high heat with extra-virgin olive oil. Add the onion, peppers, and zucchini and season to taste.

2. Cook for 3–5 minutes until slightly tender, and then add the mushrooms. Continue to cook until all is softened, stirring often. Set aside and cover to keep warm.

3. Prepare guacamole topping by mashing the avocados with lime juice.

4. Serve by scooping fajita mixture into lettuce cups and topping with guacamole.

5. Garnish with diced red onion, salsa, and cilantro (optional).

"Spaghetti" and Marinara Sauce

serves 6

Ingredients:

1 medium spaghetti squash

1 cup water

1 tablespoon extra-virgin olive oil

1 large onion, finely chopped

1 (28-ounce) jar tomato puree

1 teaspoon garlic powder

2 teaspoons dried basil

2 teaspoons dried oregano

1 teaspoon salt

½ teaspoon pepper

½ teaspoon chili powder (optional)

1 cup grated Parmesan cheese, divided (omit for Vegan option)

Directions:

1. Preheat your oven to 375° F. Slice the squash lengthwise and scoop out seeds.

2. Place squash, cut side down, in a baking dish. Add water and cover tightly with foil.

3. Bake for 20–30 minutes or until easily pierced with a fork.

4. While the squash is baking, sauté onion with extra-virgin olive oil until onion is transparent.

5. Stir in tomato puree, herbs, and seasonings. Cover and cook over low heat, stirring occasionally.

6. When the squash is ready, use your fork to scoop it out, separating the strands.

7. Stir ½ cup Parmesan cheese into the meat sauce. Serve sauce over spaghetti squash and use the remainder of the Parmesan to sprinkle on top of each dish (optional).

Shaking Beef with Ginger Sweet Potatoes

serves 2

Ingredients:

1–2 sweet potatoes, sliced in half lengthwise, then into ¼-inch-thick half-moons

2–3 tablespoons extra-virgin olive oil

1-inch piece fresh ginger, minced

12 ounces sirloin steak, cubed into 1-inch chunks

1 small red onion, sliced

2 garlic cloves, chopped

4 scallions, sliced into 1-inch pieces

3 tablespoons tamari

Splash of sake (optional)

Dash of fish sauce

Juice from 2 limes

Salt and pepper to taste

A few handfuls fresh watercress

Thai basil for serving (optional)

Directions:

1. Preheat oven to 400° F. Thoroughly toss sweet potatoes with 1 tablespoon extra-virgin olive oil and lightly salt. Place on a baking sheet and roast for 20 minutes or until tender; after the potatoes are roasted, toss with ginger.

2. While the potatoes are roasting, season chunks of steak with salt and pepper to taste. In a skillet over high heat, warm 1 tablespoon oil until hot and proceed to sear meat on all sides (while shaking the pan to continuously toss the beef) until well-browned and slightly pink in the center. Transfer meat to a plate and set aside.

3. Warm the last tablespoon oil until hot if your pan looks dry after cooking the beef. Add onions to the pan and cook until soft and translucent (around 5 minutes). Incorporate the garlic and scallions and cook for 2–3 minutes until scallions are tender. Return beef to pan and add sake, tamari, and fish sauce. Thoroughly mix and cook for 1 more minute.

4. Divide watercress between two plates and top with beef mixture and potatoes. Top with lime juice and Thai basil (optional).

Loaded Baked Sweet Potato

serves 2

Ingredients:

2 medium sweet potatoes
¾ pound lean ground beef (substitute tempeh for vegan option)
½ bell pepper, chopped
½ small onion, chopped
1 tablespoon extra-virgin olive oil
Your favorite seasonings to taste
Grated cheese, Greek yogurt, green onion, diced tomato, and cilantro to garnish (optional)

Directions:

1. Preheat oven to 450° F. Line a baking sheet with foil.

2. Pierce the sweet potatoes several times with a fork and place on the baking sheet; bake for 40 minutes or until tender.

3. Meanwhile, in a large skillet, brown the ground beef. Add the bell peppers, onions, extra-virgin olive oil, and your favorite seasonings; sauté until the onions and peppers are tender.

4. Slice the sweet potatoes open lengthwise, mash the insides and scoop the beef mixture into the middle of each sweet potato. Top with your favorite garnishes.

Loaded Mediterranean Vegan Sweet Potatoes

serves 4

Ingredients:

4 medium sweet potatoes

1 (15-ounce) can chickpeas, rinsed and drained

1 tablespoon extra-virgin olive oil

½ teaspoon each cumin, coriander, cinnamon, and paprika

¼ cup cherry tomatoes, diced

¼ cup chopped parsley, minced

2 tablespoons lemon juice

Chili garlic sauce (optional)

Garlic Herb Sauce Ingredients:

¼ cup hummus

Juice of ½ a lemon

1 teaspoon dried dill (2–3 teaspoons fresh dill)

3 cloves garlic, minced

Water or unsweetened almond milk to thin

Directions:

1. Preheat oven to 400° F and line a large baking sheet with foil.

2. Wash potatoes and cut in half, lengthwise

3. Toss chickpeas with ½ tablespoon olive oil and spices and place on the foil-lined baking sheet.

4. Lightly coat the sweet potatoes with remaining olive oil and place face down on the same baking sheet. Use an additional baking sheet if needed.

5. While the sweet potatoes and chickpeas are roasting, combine all sauce ingredients in a small bowl. Add just enough water or almond milk until you have reached a pourable consistency.

6. Prepare the topping by tossing tomato and parsley with lemon juice (and chili garlic sauce, if using) and setting aside to marinate.

7. After 25 minutes or once sweet potatoes are fork tender and the chickpeas are golden brown, remove from the oven.

8. For serving, turn potatoes flesh-side up and press down the insides. Top with chickpeas, sauce, and parsley-tomato garnish.

Easy Chicken
with Fennel Roasted Pumpkin & Vegetables

serves 3–4

Ingredients:

1 pound organic chicken drumsticks
1–2 tablespoons extra-virgin olive oil
Your favorite seasonings
1 cup celery, chopped
1 cup onion, sliced
½ pound pumpkin (cut into small cubes)
1–2 tablespoons fennel seeds

Directions:

1. Preheat oven to 375° F.

2. Toss chicken drumsticks in extra-virgin olive oil and seasonings in a baking dish and place into oven for 10 minutes.

3. Meanwhile, toss the celery, onions, and pumpkin in extra-virgin olive oil, fennel seeds, and your favorite seasonings. Add to chicken and bake for an additional 30 minutes (turn chicken over halfway through) or until chicken is cooked through and veggies are browned and tender.

Almond Falafel

makes 10 small patties

Ingredients:

1½ cups almonds
½ small zucchini
2 tablespoons sesame seeds, ground
3 tablespoons tahini
2 tablespoons lemon juice
2 tablespoons cilantro, finely chopped
2 tablespoons parsley, finely chopped
1 green onion, sliced
1 teaspoon coriander
1 teaspoon ground cumin
½ teaspoon sea salt
Dash of cayenne pepper
2–3 tablespoons coconut oil or extra-virgin olive oil

Directions:

1. Combine all ingredients (except the last) in a food processor until you have a dough-like consistency.

2. Add 2 or 3 tablespoons of coconut oil or extra-virgin olive oil to a pan over medium-low heat.

3. Form mixture into small patties and pan-cook until golden brown, 5–6 minutes per side.

4. Serve with red onions, lettuce, and tomatoes for garnish.

Roasted Sweet Potato, Quinoa, Kale, and Cranberry Salad

serves 4

Ingredients:

3 sweet potatoes, peeled and cubed
5 tablespoons extra-virgin olive oil
Pinch of salt
Freshly ground black pepper
1 cup uncooked quinoa
½ bunch Tuscan kale, thinly sliced
½ cup dried cranberries or currants
1 tablespoon balsamic vinegar
½ cup crumbled feta (omit for Vegan option)

Directions:

1. Preheat oven to 425° F. Toss sweet potatoes in 2 tablespoons extra-virgin olive oil and salt and pepper to taste. Arrange sweet potatoes on an aluminum foil–covered baking sheet and roast for 25 minutes or until tender.

2. Meanwhile, combine quinoa and 2 cups of water in a medium saucepan over high heat. Bring to a boil, then reduce heat to low and simmer, covered, for 15 minutes. Remove from heat and let sit for 5 minutes while still covered.

3. In a large bowl, combine quinoa, sweet potatoes, kale, and cranberries. In a small bowl, whisk together balsamic vinegar and remaining three tablespoons extra-virgin olive oil. Drizzle vinaigrette over salad and toss gently to combine. Fold in the feta (optional) right before serving.

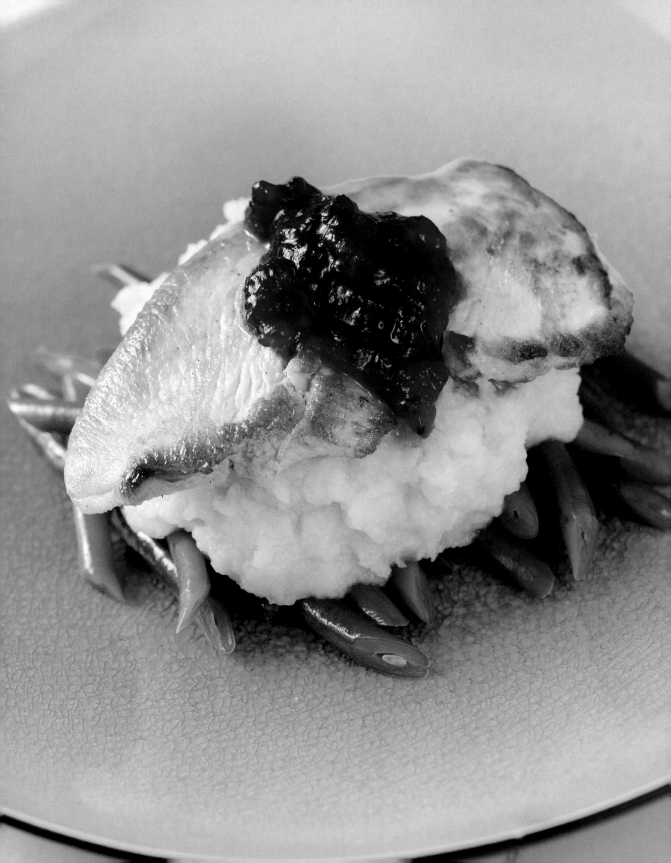

Taste of Thanksgiving Dinner

serves 3–4

Ingredients:

1 small head cauliflower
1 tablespoon extra-virgin olive oil
4 boneless, skinless turkey breast cutlets
2 cups fresh green beans
½ cup grated Parmesan cheese
2 dollops prepared cranberry sauce

Directions:

1. Chop the head of cauliflower into florets and steam for 20 minutes or until you can easily slide a fork through the florets.

2. Meanwhile, preheat a skillet over medium-high heat and add extra-virgin olive oil. Place turkey breast cutlets in hot skillet and cook, turning occasionally, for 11–13 minutes until internal temperature reaches 165° F.

3. While the turkey cutlets are cooking, steam the green beans for 5–7 minutes or until you have reached desired tenderness.

4. After the cauliflower is steamed until very tender, mash it with a fork (like you do with mashed potatoes), while adding the grated Parmesan cheese. Mash until thoroughly combined and the consistency is smooth.

5. Plate the turkey, green beans, and mashed cauliflower. Top the turkey with desired amount of cranberry sauce.

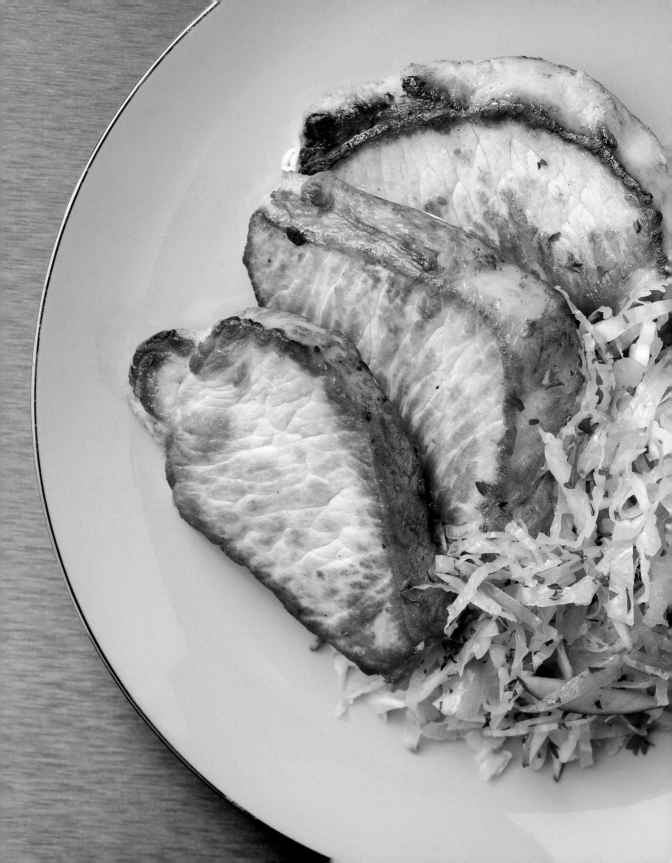

Pork Chops with Apple Cabbage Slaw

serves 4

Ingredients:

1 head cabbage, thinly sliced

1 red apple, cored and thinly sliced

2 tablespoons apple cider vinegar

4 tablespoons extra-virgin olive oil

Salt and pepper to taste

4 bone-in pork chops (around 2 pounds total)

2 teaspoons fennel seeds

2 tablespoons freshly chopped parsley

Directions:

1. Thoroughly toss cabbage, apple, vinegar, and 2 tablespoons of oil in a large bowl and season with salt and pepper. Let the slaw sit for 15–20 minutes, tossing occasionally.

2. Meanwhile, cook pork chops in a large pan or skillet using 2 tablespoons of oil. Season with salt, pepper, and fennel seeds, and cook over medium-high heat for 4 minutes on each side or until you have reached a minimum internal temperature of 145 degrees. Let the pork chops rest for 5 minutes and then serve over the slaw and garnish with more parsley.

Easy Slow Cooker Chicken Tikka Masala

serves 5-6

Ingredients:

½ cup raw cashews

2½ pounds boneless skinless chicken thighs, cut into 2-inch cubes

2 cups tomato puree

½ medium yellow onion, chopped

2 cloves garlic, minced

2½ tablespoons garam masala

2 teaspoons salt

1 teaspoon ground ginger

½ teaspoon paprika

¼ teaspoon cayenne pepper

½ cup chopped fresh cilantro for garnish

Directions:

1. Place the cashews in a bowl and cover with water. Cover with a towel or plastic wrap and set aside.

2. Place the chicken, tomato puree, onion, garlic, garam masala, salt, ginger, paprika, and cayenne pepper in a slow cooker. Cover and cook on low for 6 hours.

3. When the chicken is just about done cooking, drain the cashews and place them in a blender. Add ¼ cup of fresh water and blend the cashews into a smooth cream.

4. Stir the cashew cream into the chicken right before serving; garnish with fresh cilantro.

Turkey and Vegetable Lasagna

serves 4

Meat Sauce Ingredients:

1 pound lean ground turkey (omit turkey for vegetarian option)
1 tablespoon extra-virgin olive oil
1 large onion, diced
4 garlic cloves
7 medium tomatoes, diced
1 cup chopped basil

Meat Sauce Directions:

1. In a large skillet, cook ground turkey with extra-virgin olive oil, onion, and garlic until the turkey is medium-rare.

2. Add tomatoes to the pan and simmer on low for 15 minutes.

3. Add the basil and simmer for an additional 7–10 minutes.

*For convenience, feel free to use a store bought marinara sauce (avoid sauces with added sugar and preservatives).

Lasagna Layer Ingredients:

2 large zucchini
1 large yellow squash
1 Portobello mushroom
2 cups ricotta cheese
2 cups arugula
½ cup grated mozzarella
½ cup grated Parmigiano Reggiano

Directions:

1. Preheat the oven to 375° F.

2. Thinly slice the zucchini and yellow squash lengthwise. You will need enough strips to cover the bottom of a 9 x 13-inch baking dish and to make a second layer.

3. Slice the mushroom into thin strips.

4. Line the bottom of the baking dish with zucchini and yellow squash and cover this layer with 1 cup of meat sauce.

5. Make another layer using the mushrooms, and then layer the ricotta on top of the mushrooms, followed by another layer of zucchini and squash.

6. Make one layer of arugula on top of the zucchini and top with the remaining sauce.

7. Cover the top of the lasagna with the grated cheese. Bake uncovered for 1 hour.

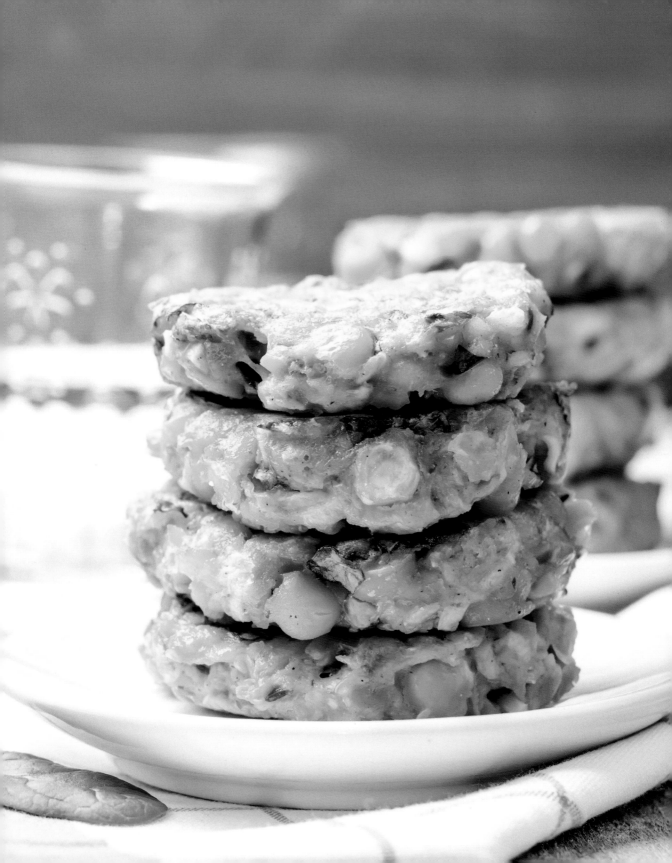

Vegan Chickpea Burgers

serves 2–3

Ingredients:

1 can chickpeas, mashed
½ red onion, diced
1 small zucchini, grated
3 tablespoons cilantro, chopped
3 tablespoons red wine vinegar
1 tablespoon sriracha sauce (optional)
2 tablespoons real peanut butter
1 teaspoon cumin
1 teaspoon garlic powder
2 teaspoons black pepper
½ teaspoon sea salt
1 cup gluten-free quick oats
2 tablespoons extra-virgin olive oil

Directions:

1. In a large bowl, mash chickpeas with a fork.

2. Add all other ingredients to the bowl and thoroughly combine. Form into 6–8 patties.

3. Grill at 400° F for 10 minutes on each side, or pan-cook in extra-virgin olive oil for 4–5 minutes on each side.

4. Serve with lettuce, tomato, onion, mustard, and avocado slices.

Six-Ingredient Apple Meatballs

serves 3–4

Ingredients:

1¼ pounds ground turkey or beef
1 cup applesauce
½ cup ground flaxseed
¼ cup almond or cashew flour
½ tablespoon sea salt
½ teaspoon cinnamon

Directions:

1. Preheat oven to 350° F.

2. Place ground meat in a mixing bowl and add applesauce, flaxseed, almond flour, salt, and cinnamon; mix until all ingredients are thoroughly combined.

3. Form mixture into 1½-inch meatballs and place on a greased baking sheet or in muffin tins to bake.

4. Bake for 30 minutes or until the outer edges start to brown.

5. Serve with salad or favorite vegetables, or on top of spaghetti squash "noodles."

Coconut Curry Shrimp with Cauliflower Rice

serves 3-4

Ingredients:

1 tablespoon coconut oil
1 onion, finely chopped
2 garlic cloves, crushed
1 teaspoon crushed ginger
1 teaspoon curry powder
½ teaspoon turmeric
1 teaspoon ground coriander
2 tablespoons freshly squeezed lemon juice
1 cup coconut milk
Sea salt and freshly ground black pepper to taste
1 pound shrimp, peeled and deveined
Cauliflower rice, cooked and ready to serve
Fresh cilantro for garnish

Directions:

1. In a hot pan, melt the coconut oil and fry the onion until golden brown.

2. Add the garlic and ginger and fry for another 10 seconds; then, add all of the spices.

3. Fry until the mixture is fragrant; then pour in the lemon juice and coconut milk and season with salt and pepper to taste.

4. Allow to simmer for 5-10 minutes until reduced slightly; then add the shrimp.

5. Allow the shrimp to cook in the sauce for 10 minutes.

6. Serve the shrimp and sauce over cauliflower rice with fresh cilantro.

Chicken Picatta

serves 3-4

Ingredients:

2 boneless, skinless chicken breasts, butterflied and then cut in half
Salt and pepper to taste
½ cup almond flour
2 tablespoons butter
3 tablespoons extra-virgin olive oil
⅓ cup fresh lemon juice
½ cup chicken stock
¼ cup capers
⅓ cup fresh parsley, chopped

Directions:

1. Season chicken with salt and pepper.

2. Dredge chicken in almond flour and shake off excess.

3. In a large skillet over medium-high heat, melt 1 tablespoon of butter with half the olive oil. When butter and oil start to sizzle, add 2 pieces of chicken and cook for 3 minutes on each side.

4. Remove and transfer to plate. Melt 1 more tablespoon of butter and add remaining olive oil. When butter and oil start to sizzle, add the other 2 pieces of chicken and brown both sides; remove the chicken and set aside.

5. Using the same pan, add the lemon juice, stock, and capers, and bring to a boil, scraping up brown bits from the pan.

6. Return all chicken to the pan and simmer for 5 minutes, adding a little more butter and oil if needed for desired consistency.

7. Remove chicken and plate; pour sauce over chicken, and garnish with parsley and fresh lemon slices.

Four-Ingredient Turmeric Scallops

serves 2

Ingredients:

1 tablespoon butter
½ pound fresh scallops
Turmeric to taste
Juice of ½ lemon

Directions:

1. Over medium heat, melt butter in a saucepan.

2. Add scallops and sprinkle with turmeric.

3. Turn each scallop over after 3–4 minutes and sprinkle other side with turmeric.

4. Cook for 3–4 more minutes or until cooked through. Top with fresh lemon juice.

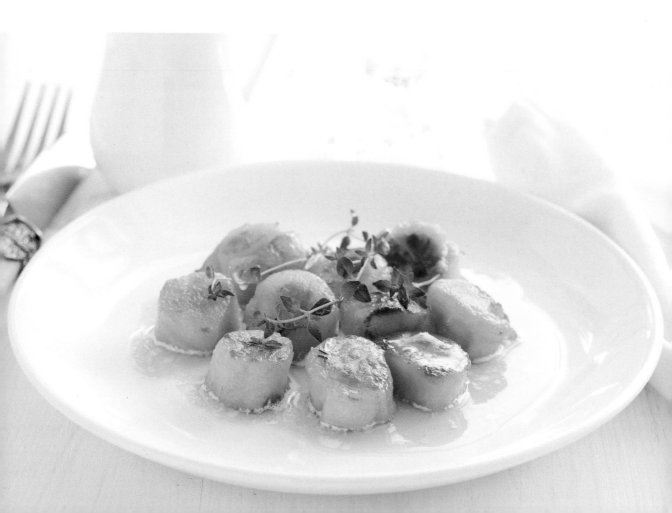

Thai Chicken Lettuce Wraps

serves 3

Ingredients:

1 tablespoon extra-virgin olive oil
1 tablespoon ginger, chopped
1 stalk lemongrass, chopped
3 red chilies, chopped
1 pound minced chicken breast
1 teaspoon fish sauce
¼ cup lemon juice
1 red onion, thinly sliced
1 cup cilantro leaves
2 tablespoons shredded basil
1 head butter lettuce

Directions:

1. Place oil in a pan over high heat and add ginger, lemongrass, and chilies; cook for 1 minute until fragrant.

2. Add the chicken and cook for 5 minutes, stirring to break up any lumps until cooked through.

3. Remove from the heat and allow to cool slightly. Combine with fish sauce and lemon juice.

4. Add the onion, cilantro, and basil. To serve, scoop mixture into lettuce cups.

Easy Crock-Pot Pulled Pork

serves 4–6

Ingredients:

2 pounds pork loin
2 tablespoons lemon juice
3 tablespoons coconut oil
7 ounces tomato paste
1 onion, chopped
1 jalapeño pepper, seeded
4 garlic cloves, minced
2 teaspoons chili powder
1 teaspoon cumin
1 teaspoon thyme
½ teaspoon cayenne pepper
½ teaspoon paprika

Directions:

1. Place all ingredients in the Crock-Pot.

2. Turn the Crock-Pot on low and cook for 5 hours.

3. Once cooked through, take two forks and shred the pork. Pair with your favorite side dishes or use in pulled pork taco lettuce wraps.

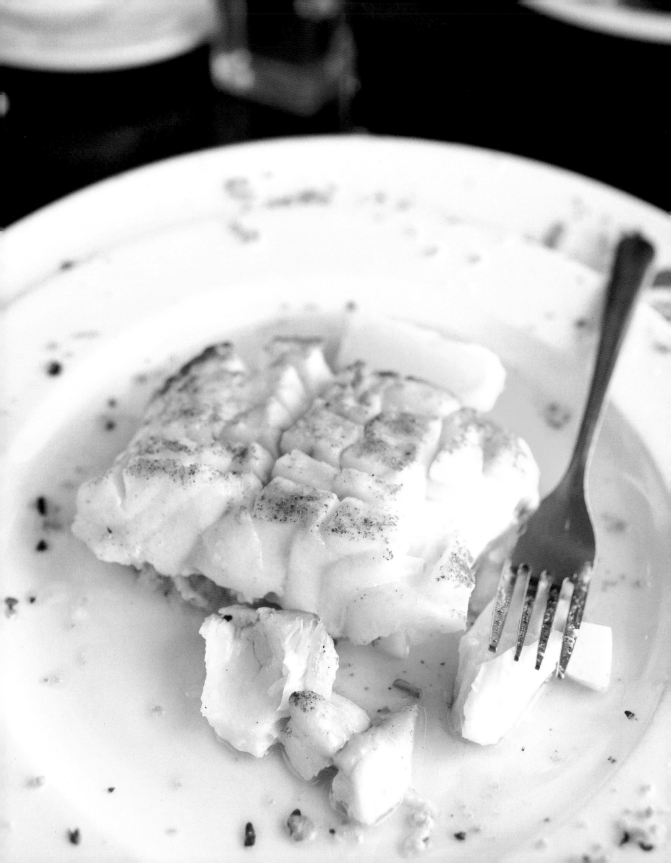

Easy Bake Lemon Butter Fish

serves 4

Ingredients:

¼ cup melted butter
4 garlic cloves, minced
Zest and juice of 1 lemon
2 tablespoons fresh parsley, minced
4 filets of cod, halibut, or rockfish
Salt and pepper to taste
1 lemon, sliced

Directions:

1. Preheat oven to 425° F.

2. In a bowl, combine the butter, garlic, lemon zest, lemon juice, and parsley; season with salt and pepper to taste.

3. Place the fish in a greased baking dish.

4. Pour the lemon butter mixture over the fish and top with fresh lemon slices.

5. Bake for 12–15 minutes, or until fish is flaky and cooked through.

6. Serve the fish topped with fresh parsley and freshly squeezed lemon juice.

Spaghetti Squash Beef Casserole

serves 3-4

Ingredients:

1 spaghetti squash
1 pound lean ground beef
½ red onion, diced
20 cherry tomatoes, halved
1 tablespoon minced garlic
2 garlic cloves, minced
2 teaspoons oregano
1 teaspoon onion powder
½ tablespoon extra-virgin olive oil
1 handful spinach, finely diced
1 whole egg

Directions:

1. Preheat oven to 400° F.

2. Cut squash in half lengthwise and remove seeds. Place on baking sheet, cut side facing down, and bake for 25 minutes.

3. While squash is baking, pan-cook ground beef over medium-high heat until cooked through; set aside.

4. While the squash is still roasting, sauté red onion, tomatoes, garlic, and seasonings with extra-virgin olive oil over medium heat. Once onions begin to turn translucent, add spinach and continue to cook for a few minutes until spinach wilts down.

5. Once squash is done roasting, remove from oven and shred the inside of the squash with a fork. Add shredded squash to the pan with sautéed vegetables. Also add the cooked meat and the egg and combine thoroughly.

6. Pour mixture in a 9 x 9-inch baking dish and cook for 15–20 minutes.

Cauliflower Fried Rice

serves 4

Ingredients:

1 (2-pound) head cauliflower, or 2 pounds already riced cauliflower (found in some stores)

4 tablespoons extra-virgin olive oil

2 large eggs, beaten

3 garlic cloves, minced

1 tablespoon finely chopped fresh ginger

4 tablespoons tamari

¼ teaspoon red pepper flakes (optional)

1 cup frozen peas and carrots

1 teaspoon rice vinegar

1 teaspoon sesame oil

1 cup chopped scallions

¼ cup chopped cashews (optional)

¼ cup chopped pineapple (optional)

Directions:

1. Grate the cauliflower in a food processor fitted with the grating disc, or on the large holes of box or hand-held grater. Set aside. (Skip this step if using premade cauliflower rice.)

2. Heat 1 tablespoon extra-virgin olive oil in large skillet over medium heat. Add the eggs and scramble until the eggs are cooked; transfer to a small plate and set aside.

3. Add 2 tablespoons extra-virgin olive oil to the pan and set over medium heat. Add garlic and ginger and cook for 3–4 minutes, stirring often, until softened.

4. Add the grated cauliflower, tamari, and red pepper flakes, if using. Cook for 3 minutes while stirring often.

5. Add the peas and carrots and continue cooking for 3–4 minutes until the cauliflower rice is slightly tender and the vegetables are warmed through.

6. Stir in the rice vinegar, sesame oil, scallions, eggs, nuts, and pineapple until thoroughly combined.

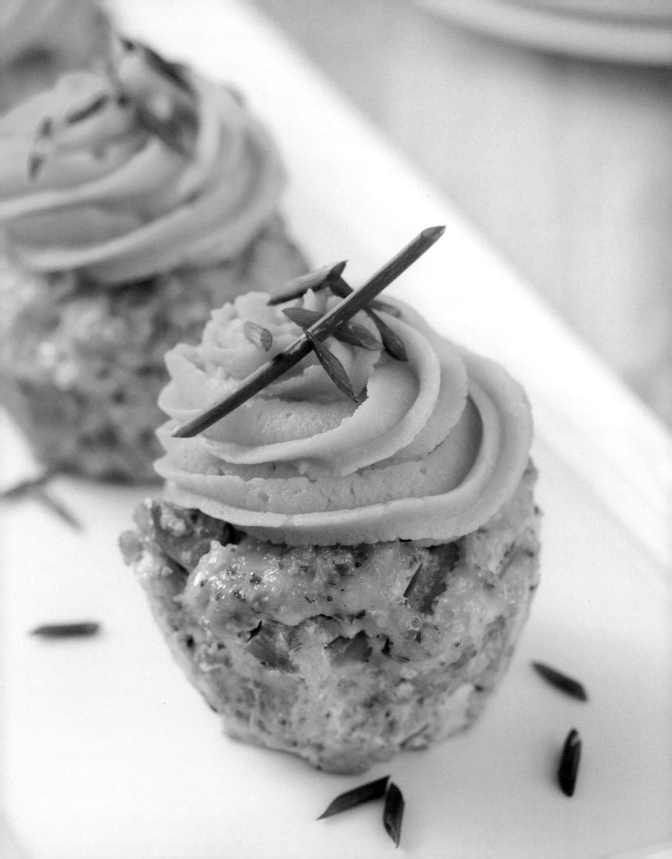

Meatloaf Muffins
with Sweet Potato Mash Topping

makes 12 "muffins"

Ingredients:

3 small sweet potatoes

2 eggs

1 small apple, diced

½ red bell pepper, diced

½ green bell pepper, diced

½ onion, diced

1½ pounds ground turkey, bison, or lean beef

¾ cup almond meal

1 teaspoon garlic powder

Black pepper to taste

½ cup tomato sauce

½ tablespoon extra-virgin olive oil to grease muffin tins

Cinnamon and nutmeg to taste

Directions:

1. Preheat oven to 350° F. Poke holes in sweet potatoes and bake for 30 minutes or until tender; set aside to cool.

2. In a large bowl, combine eggs, apple, bell peppers, and onions. Add meat, almond meal, garlic powder, black pepper, and tomato sauce; mix well with your hands until thoroughly combined.

3. Separate meatloaf mixture and divide into your greased muffin tin. Bake for 20 minutes or until meatloaf is done.

4. Meanwhile, scoop out the center of the sweet potatoes and mash with a fork (for added texture and nutrients, leave the skin on!) and combine with cinnamon and nutmeg. Scoop mashed sweet potatoes on top of muffins to serve.

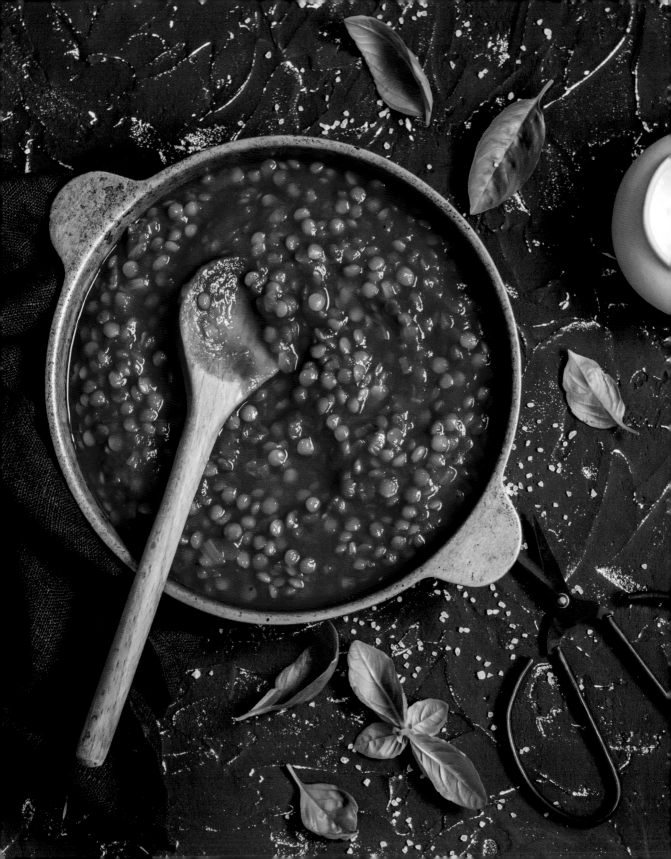

Red Lentil Bolognese

serves 4

Ingredients:

1 tablespoon extra-virgin olive oil
½ onion, diced
2 cloves garlic, minced
1 carrot, shredded
4 celery stalks, diced
4 ripe tomatoes, chopped
1 cup vegetable broth
1 cup red lentils
3 tablespoons tomato puree
1 teaspoon oregano
1 teaspoon fennel seeds
1 teaspoon black pepper
1 teaspoon chipotle powder (optional)

Directions:

1. Using a large saucepan, sauté onion, garlic, carrot, celery, and tomatoes in extra-virgin olive oil over medium heat for 5 minutes.

2. Add vegetable broth, lentils, tomato puree, and herbs/spices to pan and continue to cook over medium heat for 35–40 minutes or until lentils are soft.

3. You may serve the Bolognese by itself or over spaghetti squash noodles.

Mango Tempeh

serves 1

Ingredients:

4–6 ounces tempeh, sliced
Juice from ½ a lime
2 tablespoons white rice vinegar
1 tablespoon fresh cilantro, chopped
1 teaspoon extra-virgin olive oil

Mango Salsa Ingredients:

½ ripe mango, chopped
3 tablespoons onions, diced
3 tablespoons green peppers, diced
1 teaspoon jalapeño, diced (optional)
3 tablespoons cilantro, chopped
Juice of 1 lemon

Directions:

1. Marinate tempeh in lime juice, white rice vinegar, and cilantro for 10 minutes.

2. Meanwhile, chop all salsa ingredients and combine in a small bowl.

3. Using medium heat, sauté tempeh in a pan for 3 minutes with one teaspoon extra-virgin olive oil. Top with mango salsa.

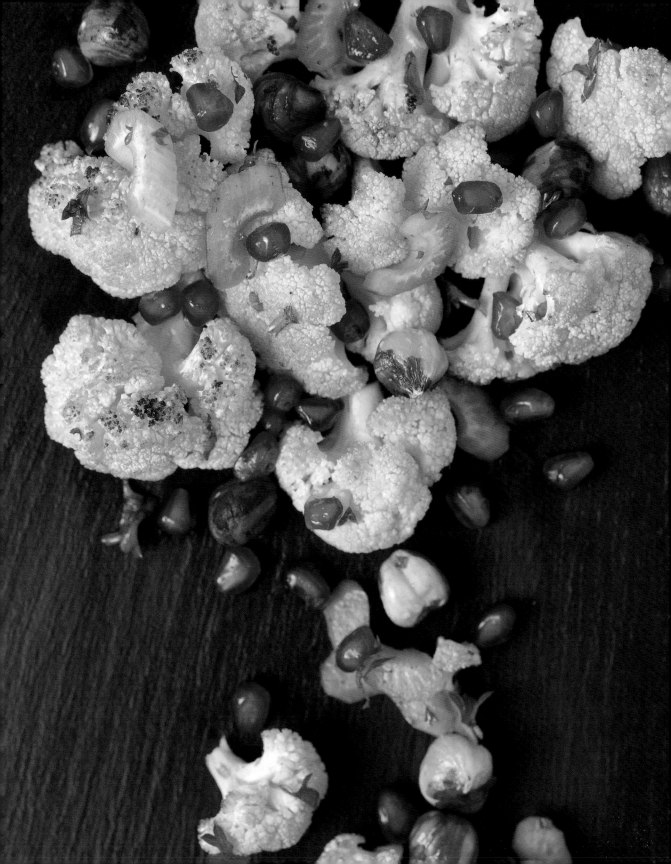

Cauliflower Pomegranate Salad

serves 3

Ingredients:

1 head cauliflower, chopped into small florets
5 tablespoons extra-virgin olive oil
5 tablespoons hazelnuts, with skins
1 large celery stalk, cut into ¼-inch slices
⅓ cup flat leaf parsley leaves
⅓ cup pomegranate arils
¼ teaspoon ground cinnamon
¼ teaspoon ground allspice
1 tablespoon sherry vinegar
1 teaspoon pure maple syrup
Salt and freshly ground black pepper

Directions:

1. Preheat oven to 425° F.

2. Mix the cauliflower florets with 3 tablespoons extra-virgin olive oil, ½ teaspoon salt, and black pepper to taste. Spread out in a roasting pan and roast on the top oven rack for 25–35 minutes, until the cauliflower is crisp and parts of it have turned golden brown.

3. Transfer to a large mixing bowl and set aside to cool.

4. Decrease the oven temperature to 325° F. Spread the hazelnuts on a baking sheet lined with parchment paper and roast for 15–17 minutes.

5. Allow the nuts to cool; coarsely chop.

6. Combine nuts with cauliflower, celery, parsley, and pomegranate arils.

7. In a small bowl or jar, combine the remaining 2 tablespoons extra-virgin olive oil with cinnamon, allspice, sherry vinegar, maple syrup, and a bit of salt and pepper to taste. Whisk together and pour over the salad.

Margherita Zucchini Pizza Boats

makes 8 mini pizzas

Ingredients:

4 zucchinis
2 tablespoons extra-virgin olive oil
2 garlic cloves, minced
¼ cup green or red pesto (optional)
1½ cups tomato sauce
1 cup shredded mozzarella
2 cups cherry tomatoes, halved
¼ cup grated Parmesan cheese
Handful of basil leaves
Your favorite seasonings

*Add ground turkey or crumbled tempeh for extra protein.

Directions:

1. Preheat oven to 350° F and lightly grease 2 medium casserole dishes with extra-virgin olive oil.

2. Cut zucchinis in half lengthwise and scrape out all seed to make room for toppings.

3. Combine the extra-virgin olive oil and garlic and brush mixture into the hollow of each zucchini boat; add your favorite seasonings.

4. Spread 1 tablespoon of the pesto in the bottom of each boat, if using, and then follow with a few tablespoons of tomato sauce. If you are adding cooked ground turkey or tempeh, add on top of the tomato sauce.

5. Sprinkle with the mozzarella and place cherry tomato halves in the cheese.

6. Sprinkle the Parmesan on top and bake in the top and bottom thirds of the oven for 20–25 minutes, rotating the dishes halfway through baking, until the cheese is browned and the zucchini has softened.

7. Garnish with fresh basil and serve.

Simple Chicken and Spinach Curry

serves 2–3

Ingredients:

1 tablespoon extra-virgin olive oil
1 pound of boneless, skinless chicken breasts, cut into 1-inch pieces
⅓ cup onion, finely chopped
1 bag of fresh spinach
2 tablespoons green curry paste
½ can unsweetened coconut milk
Cilantro for garnish

Directions:

1. In one pan, add a dash of extra-virgin olive oil and cook chicken over medium heat until cooked through.

2. In a second pan, add a dash of extra-virgin olive oil and cook the diced onion and spinach over low-medium heat for 3–4 minutes until spinach has wilted down.

3. Once your chicken is almost cooked through, add the green curry paste and coconut milk and combine; let simmer on low for 5–10 minutes, adding more coconut milk if you prefer more sauce.

4. Add the spinach and onion mixture to the pan of chicken and mix; garnish with cilantro.

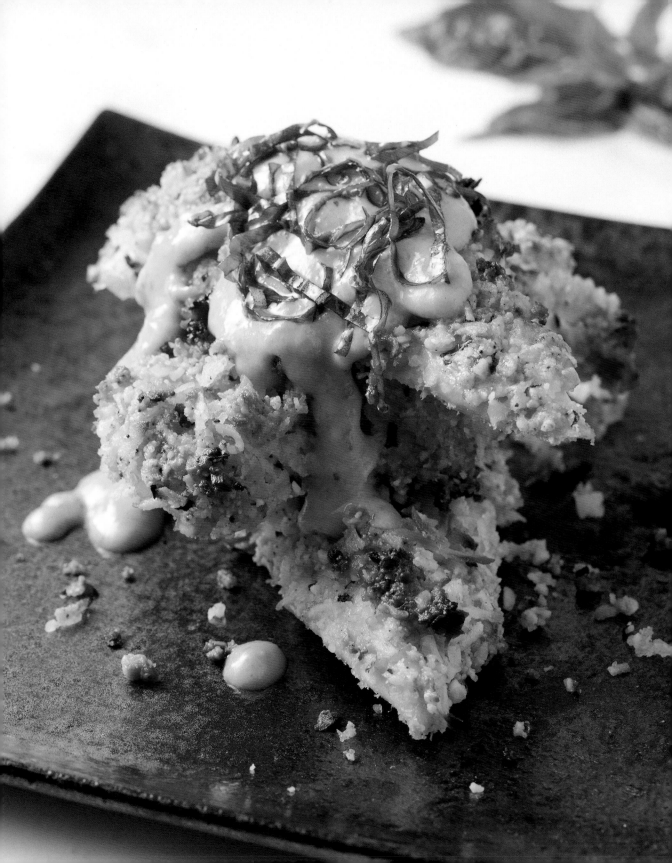

Chicken Tenders
with Mustard-Peach Dipping Sauce

serves 3–4

Chicken Tender Ingredients:

2 large eggs

½ cup macadamia nuts

½ cup unsweetened shredded coconut

½ teaspoon sea salt

4 teaspoons fresh ground pepper

¾ teaspoon garlic powder

¾ teaspoon onion powder

¼ teaspoon paprika

¼ teaspoon dried basil

1 pound chicken tenders (around 8–10 tenders)

Mustard-Peach Dipping Sauce Ingredients:

1 large peach, pitted

2 teaspoons Dijon mustard

1 teaspoon extra-virgin olive oil

Directions:

1. Preheat your oven to 375° F. Prepare a greased baking sheet.

2. In shallow dish, beat two eggs.

3. In a blender or food processor, pulse macadamia nuts until coarse.

4. In another shallow dish, combine macadamia nuts, shredded coconut, and seasonings.

5. Dip chicken tenders in egg and then into macadamia-coconut mixture to evenly coat the chicken.

6. Place coated chicken on a greased baking sheet and cook for 12 minutes. Flip the strips over and continue to cook for 10 more minutes, and then broil on high for 2 minutes until crispy.

Mustard-Peach Dip Instructions:

1. Blend all ingredients until smooth.

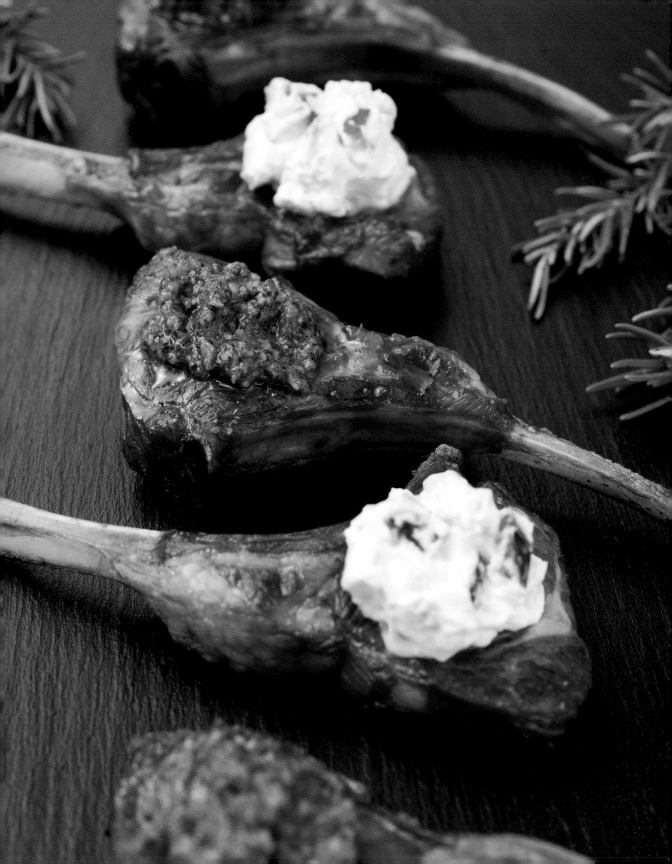

Lamb Chops
with Simple Tzatziki and Pesto Sauce

serves 5–6

Pesto Sauce Ingredients:

1½ cups fresh basil
2 tablespoons extra-virgin olive oil
½ cup pine nuts
3 garlic cloves

Lamb Ingredients:

3 pounds of lamb chops or 2 pounds of lamb steaks
1 tablespoon extra-virgin olive oil
Rosemary to taste
Salt and pepper to taste

Tzatziki Ingredients:

1 cup Greek whole milk yogurt
1 English cucumber, seeded, finely grated, and drained
2 cloves garlic, finely minced
1 teaspoon lemon zest + 1 tablespoon fresh lemon juice
2 tablespoons chopped fresh dill

Directions:

1. Place all pesto ingredients in a food processor and combine; set aside.

2. Lightly coat the lamb chops or lamb steaks with olive oil, rosemary, salt, and pepper, and grill on each side for 6–9 minutes (for lamb steaks) or 2–4 minutes (for lamb chops) or until you have cooked through to your liking.

3. While the lamb is grilling, combine all Tzatziki ingredients in a medium bowl.

4. Plate the lamb and top with both sauces.

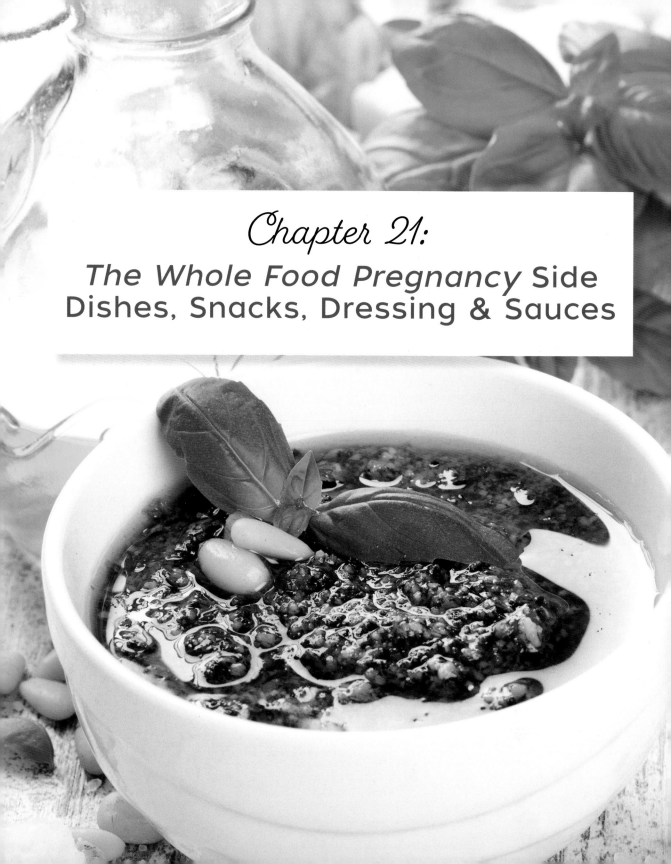

Chapter 21:
The Whole Food Pregnancy Side Dishes, Snacks, Dressing & Sauces

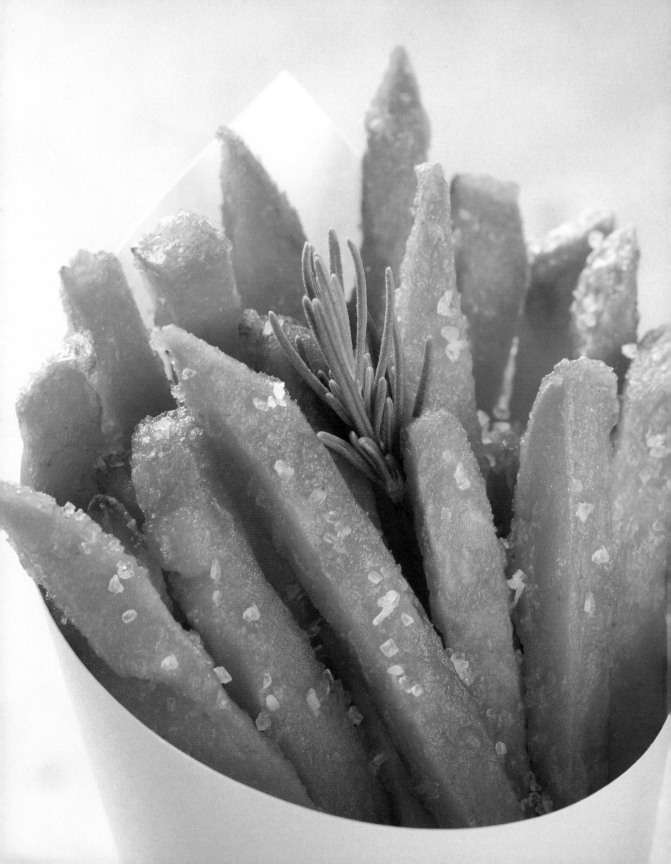

Baked Sweet Potato Fries

serves 1-2

Ingredients:

1 large sweet potato
1 tablespoon extra-virgin olive oil
Your favorite seasonings, to taste

Directions:

1. Preheat oven to 450° F.

2. Slice sweet potatoes into French fry–sized slices.

3. Toss in extra-virgin olive oil and seasonings until evenly coated.

4. Bake for 20 minutes until tender, turning over halfway through.

5. Sprinkle with sea salt (optional).

Mayo-Free Potato Salad

serves 4

Ingredients:

1 pound of small potatoes (around 1½–2-inch diameter), preferably in different colors
3 tablespoons chopped shallots
1 tablespoon Dijon mustard
1 tablespoon whole-grain mustard

1 tablespoon white wine vinegar
1 teaspoon black pepper
3 tablespoons extra-virgin olive oil
4 tablespoons chopped fresh parsley

Directions:

1. Cover the potatoes in water and boil. After the water has come to a boil, simmer until potatoes are tender (around 15 minutes).

2. Whisk together all other ingredients (except parsley) while potatoes are cooking.

3. Once potatoes are cool enough to handle, cut them in quarters and add to a large mixing bowl.

4. Evenly toss the potatoes with the mixture. Add in parsley and lightly toss again.

Seedy Dipping Crackers

serves 8

Ingredients:

1 cup gluten-free oats
¾ cup raw pumpkin seeds
⅓ cup raw sunflower seeds
⅓ cup sesame seeds
3 tablespoons chia seeds
3 tablespoons poppy seeds
1 teaspoon salt
1½ tablespoons extra-virgin olive oil
1 tablespoon pure maple syrup
¾ cup water

Directions:

1. Preheat oven to 375° F.

2. Combine oats, pumpkin seeds, sunflower seeds, sesame seeds, chia seeds, poppy seeds, and salt in a large bowl.

3. Stir oil, maple syrup, and water in a separate medium bowl and then add it to the oat mixture and combine thoroughly. Let sit for 15 minutes to thicken.

4. Form oat mixture into a ball and place on a parchment-lined baking sheet. Place a second sheet of parchment paper directly on top of the ball of dough.

5. Using a rolling pin, flatten to ⅛-inch thick and remove top layer of parchment paper.

6. Bake for 16–19 minutes until golden-brown around edges. Remove from oven and take the parchment paper (with cracker) off the baking sheet; line the baking sheet with a new piece of parchment paper.

7. Flip the cracker over onto the new piece of parchment paper that is now lining the baking sheet and discard the old piece of parchment paper.

8. Bake for an additional 15–20 minutes until edges are golden-brown; remove from the oven, and cool. Break into cracker sized pieces and pair with your favorite dip.

Creamy Cucumber Salad

serves 2

Ingredients:

½ cup plain almond or coconut yogurt
1 green onion, chopped
Black pepper to taste
1 tablespoon fresh dill, chopped, or ½ teaspoon dried dill
1 clove of garlic, minced
½ cup cucumber, thinly sliced
1 tablespoon red onion, sliced

Directions:

1. Combine yogurt with green onion, pepper, dill, and garlic.

2. Add cucumbers and red onion and toss until evenly coated.

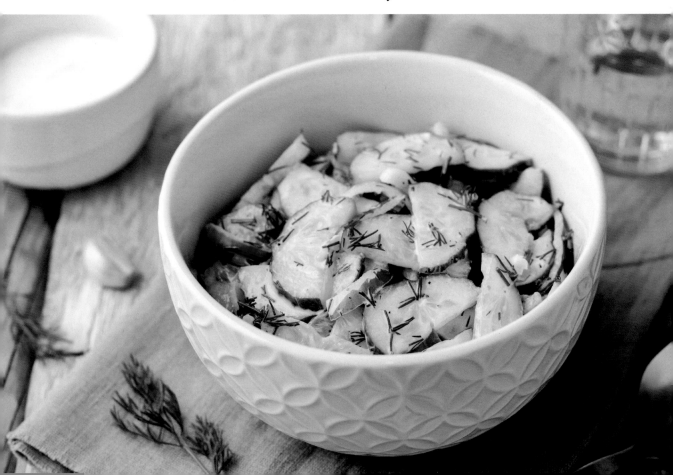

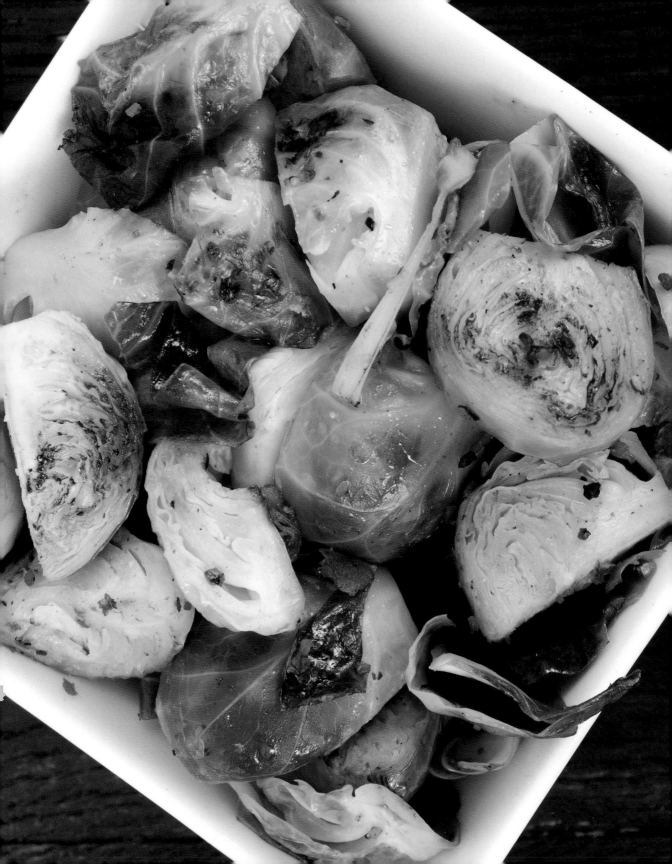

Not Your Regular Brussels Sprouts

serves 1

Ingredients:

6 medium-large Brussels sprouts
1 teaspoon extra-virgin olive oil
Garlic powder to taste
Black pepper to taste
Freshly squeezed lemon

Directions:

1. Heat extra-virgin olive oil in a pan over medium heat and evenly distribute the oil throughout the surface of the pan.

2. Place the Brussels sprouts flat side down in the oil and sprinkle with garlic and black pepper.

3. Cook for 5 minutes or until the flat side of the sprouts are browned and turn the sprouts over to the round side. Add a bit more oil if needed.

4. Lower the heat to low and cook on the round side of the sprouts for 7 minutes with a cover over the pan.

5. Plate and top with freshly squeezed lemon juice.

Parmesan Roasted Fennel

serves 2-3

Ingredients:

1 large fennel bulb, stems removed, and quartered
2 tablespoons grated Parmesan cheese
1 tablespoon extra-virgin olive oil

Directions:

1. Preheat your oven to 400° F.

2. Boil or steam the quartered fennel until tender; toss in extra-virgin olive oil.

3. Roast for 10 minutes; sprinkle with Parmesan cheese and roast for 2 additional minutes.

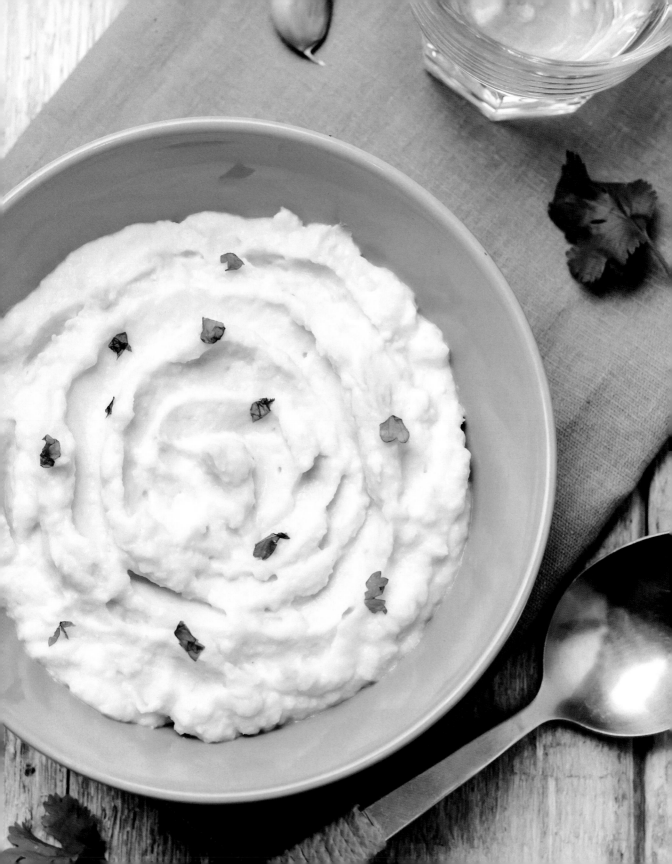

Mashed Cauliflower

serves 4

Ingredients:

1 head of cauliflower
½ cup grated Parmesan cheese

Directions:

1. Chop cauliflower and steam until extremely tender.

2. Using a potato masher or fork, mash into a mashed potato-like texture.

3. Add grated Parmesan and thoroughly combine.

Mushroom Stroganoff

serves 6–8

Mushroom Ingredients:

4 cups mushrooms, sliced
3 cloves garlic, minced
½ yellow onion, thinly sliced
3 tablespoons extra-virgin olive oil
3 tablespoons tamari
¼ cup white wine

Stroganoff Sauce Ingredients:

2 tablespoons extra-virgin olive oil
1 tablespoon sun-dried tomatoes
1 tablespoon paprika
½ cup vegetable stock
½ cup cashews
1 teaspoon rosemary
1 teaspoon thyme
1 teaspoon black pepper

Directions:

1. Toss sliced mushrooms, garlic, and onion together in the olive oil and tamari. Set aside and marinate for 10–15 minutes.

2. Pan-cook mushroom mixture in a skillet over medium heat until tender; add wine and simmer for 5 minutes.

3. For the sauce, in a food processor or blender, combine extra-virgin olive oil, sun-dried tomatoes, paprika, vegetable stock, cashews, rosemary, thyme, and pepper until smooth.

4. Transfer into the pan with mushrooms and continue to simmer until sauce thickens.

5. Serve on its own as a side dish or as a protein topping.

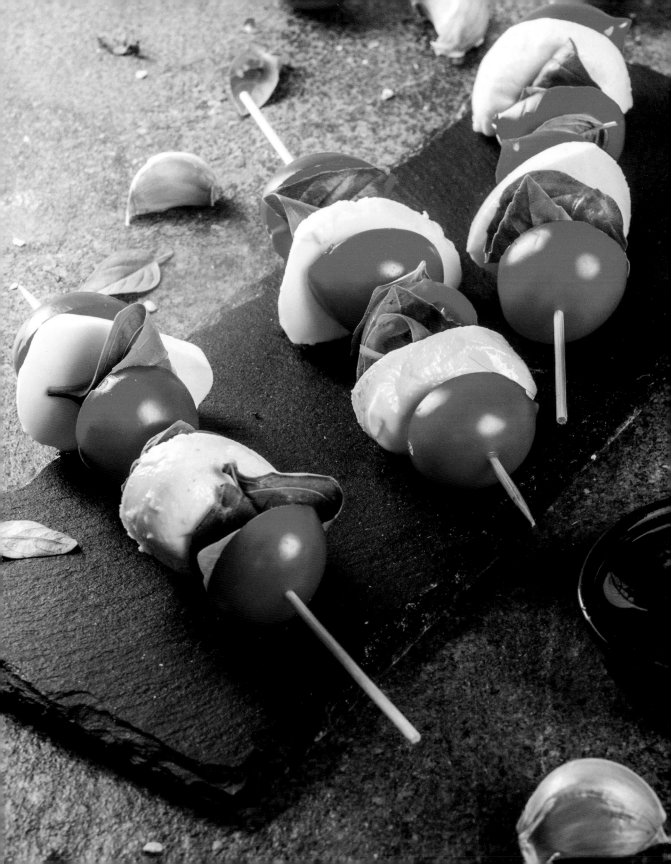

Caprese Skewers

serves 3

Ingredients:

½ cup balsamic vinegar
2 tablespoons honey
1 cup mozzarella cheese balls
1 cup cherry tomatoes, halved
½ cup fresh basil leaves
3 wooden skewers (optional)

Directions:

1. Stir balsamic vinegar and honey together in a small saucepan and place over high heat. Bring to a boil, reduce heat to low, and simmer until the vinegar mixture has reduced down to a syrup, about 10 minutes. Set the balsamic reduction aside to cool.

2. Place the cheese, tomato, and basil leaves on the skewer in desired arrangement.

3. Plate the caprese skewers and drizzle with balsamic reduction.

Sweet & Nutty Avocado

serves 1

Ingredients:

½ avocado
Drizzle of honey or agave
½ tablespoon sunflower seeds

Directions:

1. Remove pit from half of an avocado.

2. Lightly drizzle with honey or agave.

3. Fill the pit hole with sunflower seeds and lightly drizzle again with your sweetener of choice.

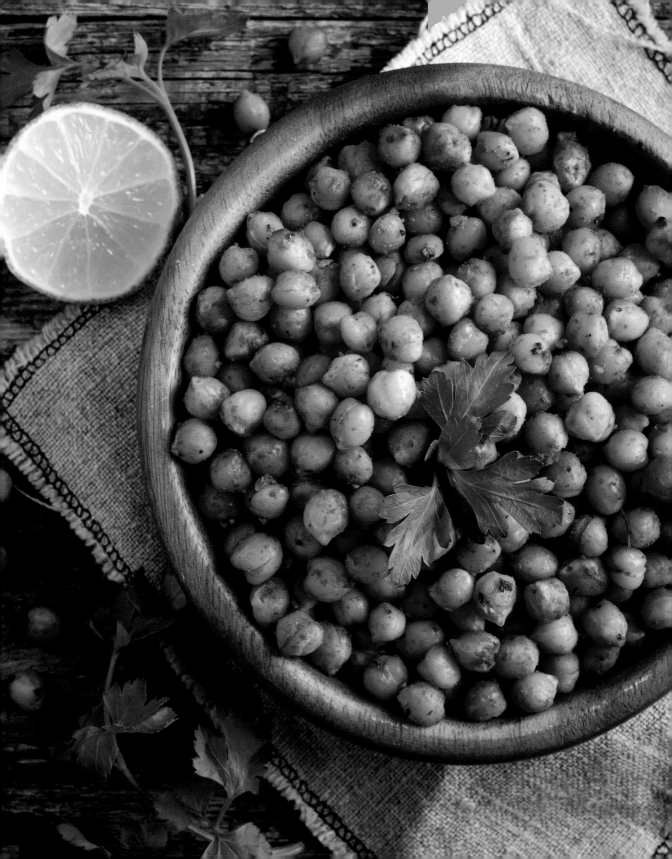

Salt and Vinegar Chickpeas

serves 4

Ingredients:

2 cups canned chickpeas
3–4 cups white vinegar
1 teaspoon coarse sea salt
2 teaspoons extra-virgin olive oil

Directions:

1. Preheat oven to 400° F.

2. Line a baking sheet with tin foil or parchment paper.

3. Place chickpeas and vinegar in a medium-sized pot; add a dash of sea salt.

4. Bring to a boil and then remove from heat; let sit in pot for 30 minutes.

5. Drain chickpeas and place on lined baking sheet. Drizzle with extra-virgin olive oil and sea salt; hand toss until evenly coated.

6. Roast for 30–40 minutes, flipping once halfway through. Check the chickpeas at 25 minutes to make sure they are not darkening beyond a golden-brown color.

Kale Chips

serves 2–3

Ingredients:

3 cups curly kale
1 tablespoon extra-virgin olive oil
A few dashes of salt to taste

Directions:

1. Preheat oven to 350° F.

2. Wash, dry, and chop kale into chip-sized pieces.

3. Drizzle extra-virgin olive oil over the kale and use your hands to evenly massage the oil into all leaves.

4. Bake for 10–12 minutes or until edges are lightly browned, and lightly salt.

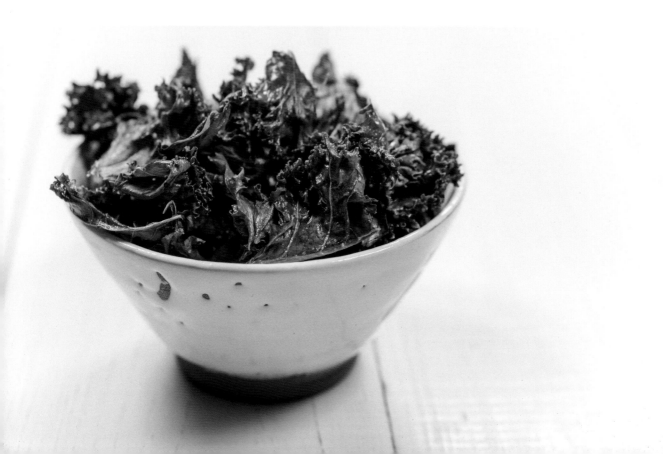

Beet Chips

serves 2

Ingredients:

3 large beets, rinsed and cleaned

1 tablespoon extra-virgin olive oil

Sea salt and black pepper to taste (optional)

2–3 sprigs rosemary, roughly chopped (optional)

Directions:

1. Place oven rack in the center of the oven and preheat oven to 375° F.

2. Thinly slice the beets (they may curl a little when sliced thinly enough).

3. Toss the beet slices in extra-virgin olive oil and seasonings until evenly coated. Lightly coat the baking sheet with extra-virgin olive oil as well to prevent sticking.

4. Arrange the beets in a single layer on the baking sheet so they are not touching each other.

5. Bake for 15–18 minutes or until crispy and slightly brown.

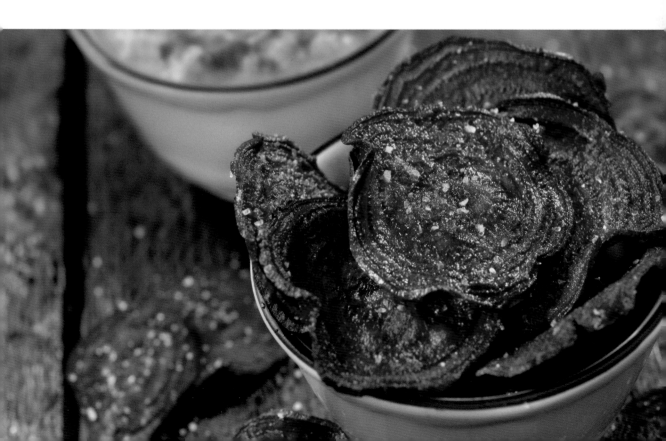

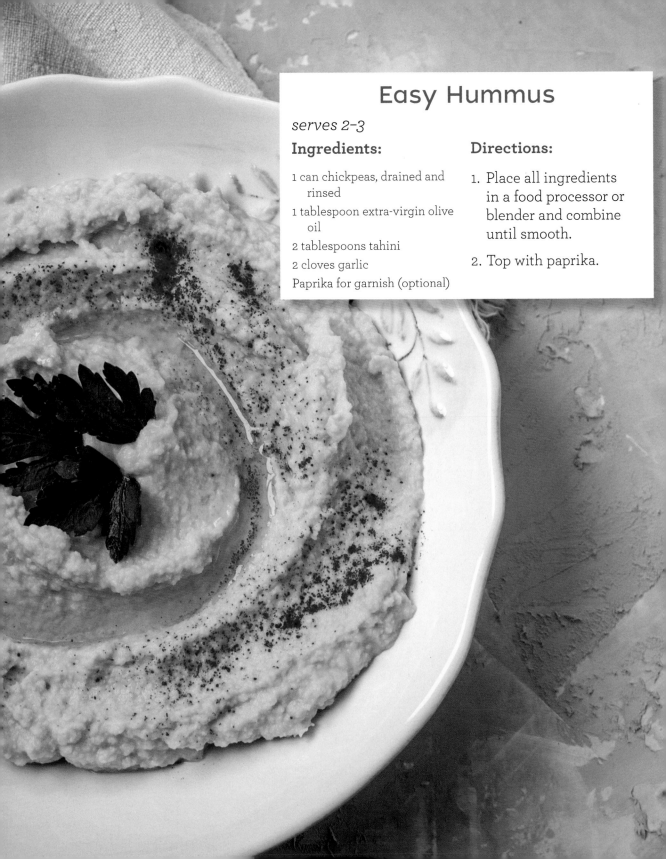

Easy Hummus

serves 2–3

Ingredients:

1 can chickpeas, drained and rinsed

1 tablespoon extra-virgin olive oil

2 tablespoons tahini

2 cloves garlic

Paprika for garnish (optional)

Directions:

1. Place all ingredients in a food processor or blender and combine until smooth.

2. Top with paprika.

Tzatziki Spread

serves 4

Ingredients:

1 cup Greek whole milk yogurt
1 English cucumber, diced
2 cloves garlic, minced
1 teaspoon lemon zest + 1 tablespoon fresh lemon juice
2 tablespoons fresh dill, chopped
1 tablespoon fresh mint, finely chopped
Sea salt and pepper to taste (optional)

Directions:

1. In a medium mixing bowl combine all ingredients.

2. Serve cold with favorite vegetables.

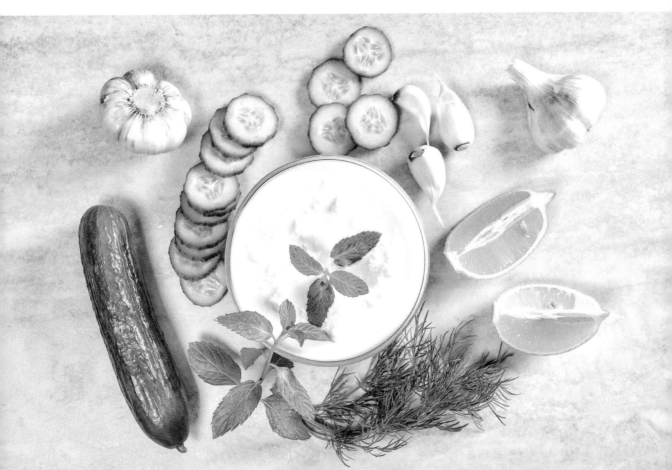

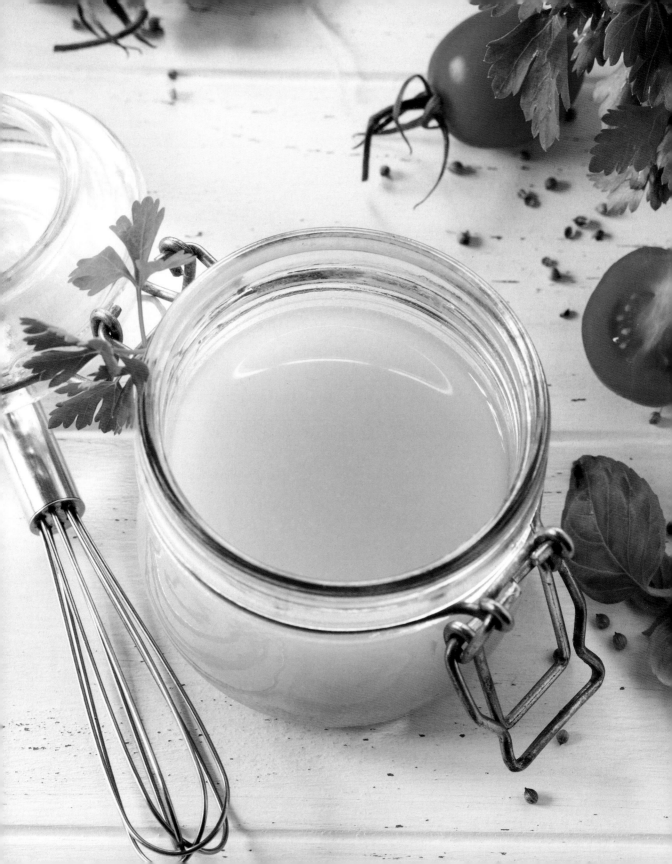

DRESSINGS AND SAUCES

Classic Vinaigrette

Ingredients:

1 part balsamic vinegar
2 parts extra-virgin olive oil
1 garlic clove
Dash of honey
Black pepper to taste

Directions:

1. Smash garlic clove with back of a knife and add to all other ingredients; whisk together.

Lemon Vinaigrette

Ingredients:

¼ cup red wine vinegar
2 tablespoons Dijon mustard
1 clove garlic, minced
1 teaspoon dried oregano
¼ teaspoon ground black pepper
½ cup olive oil
2 tablespoons fresh lemon juice

Directions:

1. Whisk vinegar, mustard, garlic, oregano, and black pepper in a small bowl until blended.

2. Drizzle in oil, whisking until blended.

3. Beat lemon juice into the mixture.

Simple Dijon

Ingredients:

1½ tablespoons white wine or cider vinegar
1 tablespoon Dijon mustard
1 lemon, juiced
1 shallot

Directions:

1. Dice shallot and add to all other ingredients; whisk together.

Raspberry Vinaigrette

Ingredients:

2 tablespoons raspberry vinegar
Freshly ground pepper, to taste
⅓ cup extra-virgin olive oil

Directions:

1. Whisk vinegar and pepper in a small bowl. Slowly whisk in oil.

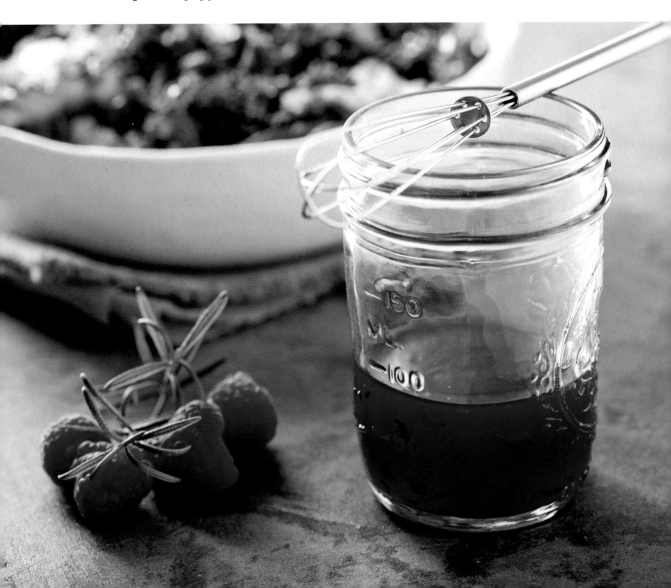

Creamy Tahini-Honey Dressing

Ingredients:

½ cup lemon juice

⅓ cup extra-virgin olive oil

⅓ cup tahini

2 tablespoons honey (or real maple syrup)

2 cloves garlic, minced

Freshly ground pepper, to taste

Directions:

1. Blend all ingredients together until mixture is creamy and smooth.

Apple Cider Vinaigrette

Ingredients:

1 part cider vinegar
1 part apple juice
2 parts extra-virgin olive oil
Black pepper to taste
Cayenne pepper to taste
Ground cinnamon to taste

Directions:

1. Whisk all ingredients together.

Smooth Tomato and Goat Cheese

Ingredients:

¼ cup crumbled goat cheese
2 tablespoons white wine vinegar
¼ cup extra-virgin olive oil
2 plum tomatoes, seeded and
    chopped
½ teaspoon salt
Freshly ground pepper, to taste
1 tablespoon chopped fresh tarragon
    (optional)

Directions:

1. Blend all ingredients together until mixture is creamy and smooth (makes 1 cup and can be refrigerated for up to 3 days).

Lime and Cilantro Vinaigrette

Ingredients:

1 cup packed cilantro
½ cup extra-virgin olive oil
¼ cup lime juice
¼ cup orange juice
½ teaspoon pepper
Pinch of minced garlic

Directions:

1. Blend all ingredients together until mixture is creamy and smooth (makes 1 cup and can be refrigerated for up to 3 days).

Healthy Honey Mustard

Ingredients:

1 clove garlic, minced

1 tablespoon white wine vinegar

1½ teaspoons Dijon mustard (coarse or smooth)

½ teaspoon honey

Freshly ground pepper, to taste

⅓ cup extra-virgin olive oil

Directions:

1. Whisk garlic, vinegar, mustard, honey, and pepper in a small bowl. Slowly whisk in oil.

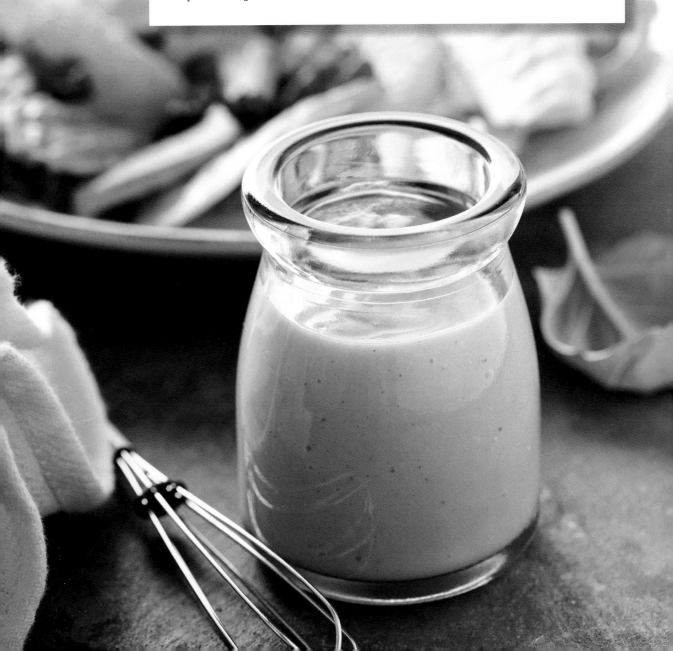

Fancy Cilantro and Basil Citrus

Ingredients:

¼ cup chopped basil
¼ cup chopped cilantro
2 tablespoons lime juice
2 tablespoons orange juice
1 teaspoon honey
1 teaspoon grated ginger
½ teaspoon lime zest
Dash of pepper
2 tablespoons extra-virgin olive oil

Directions:

1. Blend or puree all ingredients (except extra-virgin olive oil)

2. Once those ingredients are blended, continue to incorporate the oil, using the blender or food processor.

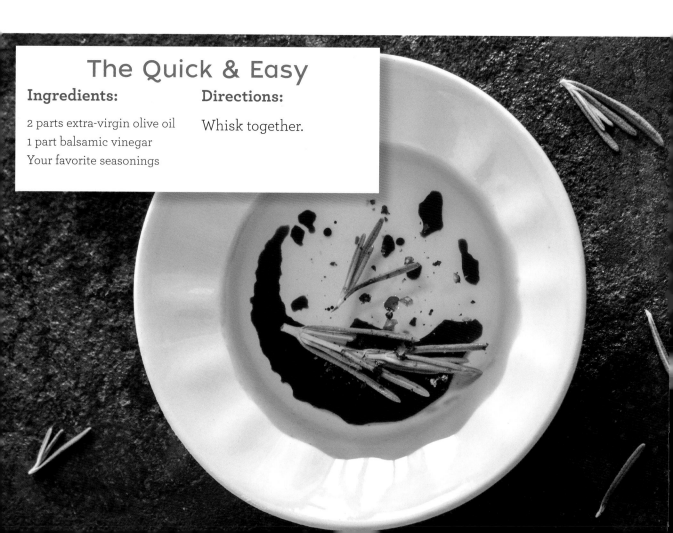

The Quick & Easy

Ingredients:

2 parts extra-virgin olive oil
1 part balsamic vinegar
Your favorite seasonings

Directions:

Whisk together.

Asian Sesame Vinaigrette

Ingredients:

¼ cup orange juice

¼ cup rice vinegar

2 tablespoons tamari

1 tablespoon toasted sesame oil

1 tablespoon honey or real maple syrup

1 teaspoon fresh ginger, finely grated

Directions:

1. Blend all ingredients together until mixture is creamy and smooth (makes ½ cup and can be refrigerated for up to 7 days).

Pesto

Ingredients:

1½ cups fresh basil leaves (packed)

¼ teaspoon freshly ground black pepper

¼ cup freshly grated Parmigiano-Reggiano (optional)

2 tablespoons pine nuts or walnuts

1 teaspoon minced garlic

½ cup extra-virgin olive oil

Directions:

1. Using a food processor or blender, combine the basil and pepper and process/blend for a few seconds until the basil is chopped.

2. Add the cheese, nuts, and garlic and while the processor is running, add the oil in a thin, steady stream until you have reached a smooth consistency.

Mango Salsa

Ingredients:

1 mango, peeled and diced

½ cup cucumber, peeled and diced

1 tablespoon finely chopped jalapeño (optional)

⅓ cup diced red onion

1 tablespoon lime juice

⅓ cup roughly chopped cilantro leaves

Directions:

1. Combine all ingredients and mix well.

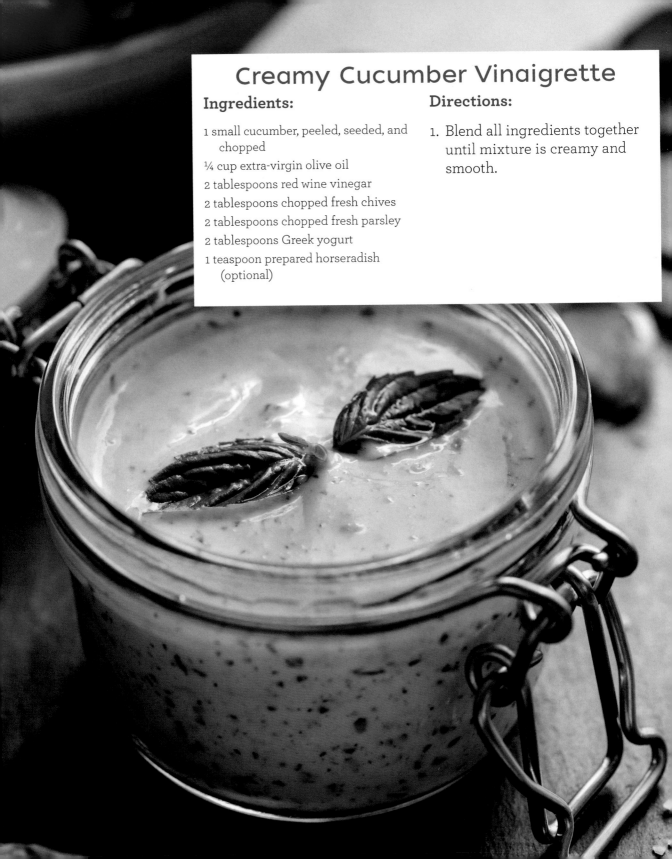

Creamy Cucumber Vinaigrette

Ingredients:

1 small cucumber, peeled, seeded, and chopped

¼ cup extra-virgin olive oil

2 tablespoons red wine vinegar

2 tablespoons chopped fresh chives

2 tablespoons chopped fresh parsley

2 tablespoons Greek yogurt

1 teaspoon prepared horseradish (optional)

Directions:

1. Blend all ingredients together until mixture is creamy and smooth.

Horseradish Cream Sauce

Ingredients:

1 cup Greek yogurt
¼ cup grated fresh horseradish
1 tablespoon Dijon mustard
1 teaspoon white wine vinegar
¼ teaspoon freshly ground black pepper

Directions:

1. Place all of the ingredients into a medium mixing bowl and whisk until the mixture is smooth and creamy.

2. Refrigerate for at least 4 hours to allow flavors to meld.

Chimichurri Sauce

Ingredients:

1 bunch parsley, finely chopped
1 bunch cilantro, finely chopped
3 tablespoons capers, finely chopped
2 garlic cloves, minced
1½ tablespoons red wine vinegar
½ teaspoon red pepper flakes
½ teaspoon ground black pepper
½ cup extra-virgin olive oil

Directions:

1. Put the parsley, cilantro, capers, and garlic in a medium mixing bowl and toss to combine.

2. Add the vinegar, both peppers, and stir.

3. Pour in the olive oil and mix until well combined; let sit for 30 minutes so that the flavors blend.

White Wine Sauce

Ingredients:

½ cup chicken broth
¼ cup white wine
Juice from ½ a lemon
1 tablespoon shallot, minced
1 clove garlic, minced
1 tablespoon butter
1 tablespoon extra-virgin olive oil
Black pepper, to taste

Directions:

1. Combine all ingredients in pan and use as a simmer sauce.

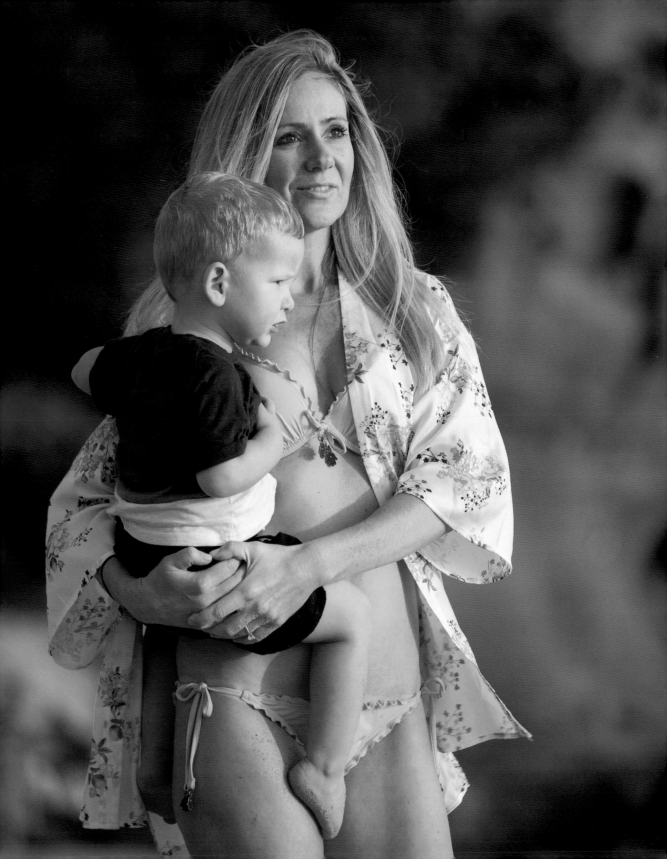

Reflection

I hope you have had a wonderful, healthy pregnancy journey and that the information found in *The Whole Food Pregnancy Plan* has benefited you. As I sit here reflecting on my own journey of prenatal nutrition, postpartum weight loss, and breastfeeding, my son is now three years old. The most important piece of insight I can pass on at this point has nothing to do with nutrition: Enjoy the fleeting time you have with your baby. In the beginning, the constant cycle of feeding, washing, rinsing, and repeating seems to be endless; the sun comes up and the sun goes down with the repetitious routine resulting in what seems to be an endless groundhog day.

There will be a day (and it will come quickly) that your baby will no longer be a baby. In the first days of struggling with a newborn while keeping my nutrition and workout regimen intact and maintaining a milk supply, things were overwhelming.

I was baffled by the statement "it goes so fast" and naively wished at some points that Alex could grow up sooner rather than later. He and I attended our last "mommy and me" lesson in August, 2017, so now I will be sitting on the sidelines and watching him grow into the little boy he has already become. While I am excited about his progress, I now miss our attached time together.

I don't mean to take away from the importance of your nutrition because it is so critical, but the *most* important aspect of this journey is spending quality time with your baby and being a positive example. To give your best to your child, you have to maintain your own health, wellness, self-care, energy, and positivity. I truly hope *The Whole Food Pregnancy Plan* plays some role in helping you be the best version of yourself for your little one.

References

Abbaspour, N., R. Hurrell, and R. Kelishadi. "Review on iron and its importance for human health." NCBI. November 27, 2013. Accessed September 06, 2017. https://www.ncbi.nlm.nih.gov/pmc/articles/PMC3999603/#__ffn_sectitle.

Al Emadi, S., and M. Hammoudeh. "Vitamin D study in pregnant women and their babies." NCBI. November 01, 2013. Accessed September 11, 2017. https://www.ncbi.nlm.nih.gov/pmc/articles/PMC3991049/.

American Psychological Association, "What is postpartum depression and anxiety?" American Psychological Association. Accessed September 11, 2017. http://www.apa.org/pi/women/resources/reports/postpartum-depression.aspx.

Bell, JM, and PK Lundberg. "Effects of a commercial soy lecithin preparation on development of sensorimotor behavior and brain biochemistry in the rat." NCBI. January 1985. Accessed September 10, 2017. https://www.ncbi.nlm.nih.gov/pubmed/4038491.

Bender, DA. "Vitamin B6 requirements and recommendations." NCBI. May 1989. Accessed September 29, 2017. https://www.ncbi.nlm.nih.gov/pubmed/2661220.

Bodnar, Lisa M., and Katherine L. Wisner. "Nutrition and Depression: Implications for Improving Mental Health among Childbearing-Aged Women." Biological psychiatry. November 01, 2005. Accessed September 13, 2017. https://www.ncbi.nlm.nih.gov/pmc/articles/PMC4288963/.

Brown, A., and V. Harries. "Infant Sleep and Night Feeding Patterns During Later Infancy: Association with Breastfeeding Frequency, Daytime Complementary Food Intake, and Infant Weight." Mary Anne Liebert, Inc. Publishers. June 09, 2015. Accessed September 29, 2017. http://online.liebertpub.com/doi/10.1089/bfm.2014.0153.

Chausmer, AB. "Zinc, insulin and diabetes." NCBI. April 1998. Accessed September 29, 2017. https://www.ncbi.nlm.nih.gov/pubmed/9550453.

Chavarro, J., J. Rich-Edwards, B. Rosner, and W. Willett. "A prospective study of dietary carbohydrate quantity and quality in relation to risk of ovulatory infertility." NCBI. September 19, 2007. Accessed September 13, 2017. https://www.ncbi.nlm.nih.gov/pmc/articles/PMC3066074/.

Chavarro, JE, JW Rich-Edwards, BA Rosner, and WC Willett. "Iron intake and risk of ovulatory infertility." NCBI. November 2006. Accessed September 19, 2017. https://www.ncbi.nlm.nih.gov/pubmed/17077236.

Coletta, J., S. Bell, and A. Roman. "Omega-3 Fatty Acids and Pregnancy." NCBI. October 2010. Accessed September 10, 2017. https://www.ncbi.nlm.nih.gov/pmc/articles/PMC3046737/.

De Punder, K., and L. Pruimboom. "The Dietary Intake of Wheat and other Cereal Grains and Their Role in Inflammation." NCBI. March 12, 2015. Accessed September 10, 2017. https://www.ncbi.nlm.nih.gov/pmc/articles/PMC3705319/#!po=59.5238

Dosman, C., M. Witmans, and L. Zwaigenbaum. "Iron's role in paediatric restless legs syndrome – a review." NCBI. April 2012. Accessed September 29, 2017. https://www.ncbi.nlm.nih.gov/pmc/articles/PMC3381661/.

Durlach, J . "New data on the importance of gestational Mg deficiency." NCBI. December 2004. Accessed September 29, 2017. https://www.ncbi.nlm.nih.gov/pubmed/15637217.

Feskanich, D., WC Willett, MJ Stampfer, and GA Colditz. "Milk, dietary calcium, and bone fractures in women: a 12-year prospective study." NCBI. June 1997. Accessed September 11, 2017. https://www.ncbi.nlm.nih.gov/pmc/articles/PMC1380936/.

Ganmaa, D., and A. Sato. "The possible role of female sex hormones in milk from pregnant cows in the development of breast, ovarian and corpus uteri cancers." NCBI. 2005. Accessed September 30, 2017. https://www.ncbi.nlm.nih.gov/pubmed/16125328.

Gao, J., J. Wu, XN Zhao, WN Zhang, YY Zhang, and ZX Zhang. "[Transplacental neurotoxic effects of monosodium glutamate on structures and functions of specific brain areas of filial mice]." NCBI. February 01, 1994. Accessed September 02, 2017. https://www.ncbi.nlm.nih.gov/pubmed/8085168.

Gaskins, A., S. Mumford, J. Chavarro, C. Zhang, A. Pollack, J. Wactawski-Wende, N. Perkins, and E. Schisterman. "The Impact of Dietary Folate Intake on Reproductive Function in Premenopausal Women: A Prospective Cohort Study." NCBI. September 26, 2012. Accessed September 20, 2017. https://www.ncbi.nlm.nih.gov/pmc/articles/PMC3458830/.

"Global, regional, and national levels of maternal mortality, 1990-2015: a systematic analysis for the Global Burden of Disease Study 2015." NCBI. October 08, 2016. Accessed September 04, 2017. https://www.ncbi.nlm.nih.gov/pubmed/?term=GBD%202015%20Maternal%20Mortality%20Collaborators%5BCorporate%20Author%5D.

Gomez Arango, LF, HL Barrett, LK Callaway, and MD Nitert. "Probiotics and pregnancy." NCBI. January 02, 2015. Accessed September 05, 2017. https://www.ncbi.nlm.nih.gov/pubmed/25398206.

Haji Seid Javadi, E., F. Salehi, and O. Mashrabi. "Comparing the Effectiveness of Vitamin B6 and Ginger in Treatment of Pregnancy-Induced Nausea and Vomiting." NCBI. October 22, 2013. Accessed September 13, 2017. https://www.ncbi.nlm.nih.gov/pmc/articles/PMC3819920/.

Halldorsson, TI, M. Strøm, SB Petersen, and SF Olsen. "Intake of artificially sweetened soft drinks and risk of preterm delivery: a prospective cohort study in 59,334 Danish pregnant women." NCBI. September 2010. Accessed September 24, 2017. https://www.ncbi.nlm.nih.gov/pubmed/20592133.

Hanson, LA. "Breastfeeding provides passive and likely long-lasting active immunity." NCBI. December 1998. Accessed October 01, 2017. https://www.ncbi.nlm.nih.gov/pubmed/9892025.

Harvard Health. "What meditation can do for your mind, mood, and health." Harvard Health. Accessed September 12, 2017. https://www.health.harvard.edu/staying-healthy/what-meditation-can-do-for-your-mind-mood-and-health-.

Heitlinger, LA. "Enzymes in mother's milk and their possible role in digestion." NCBI. 1983. Accessed October 01, 2017. https://www.ncbi.nlm.nih.gov/pubmed/6196470.

Herring, Sharon, and Emily Oken. "Obesity and Diabetes in Mothers and Their Children: Can We Stop the Intergenerational Cycle?" NCBI. February 01, 2011. Accessed September 04, 2017. https://www.ncbi.nlm.nih.gov/pmc/articles/PMC3191112/pdf/nihms327612.pdf

Jackson, LS, and K. Lee. "The effect of dairy products on iron availability." NCBI. September 29, 2009. Accessed September 13, 2017. https://www.ncbi.nlm.nih.gov/pubmed/1581006.

Jaikatis, BM, and PW Denning. "Human breast milk and the gastrointestinal innate immune system." NCBI. June 2014. Accessed September 29, 2017. https://www.ncbi.nlm.nih.gov/pubmed/24873841.

Jarjou, L. MA, Y. Sawo, G. Goldberg, M. Laskey, T. Cole, and A. Prentice. "Unexpected long-term effects of calcium supplementation in pregnancy on maternal bone outcomes in women with a low calcium intake: a follow-up study1,2,3." NCBI. June 13, 2013. Accessed September 06, 2017. https://www.ncbi.nlm.nih.gov/pmc/articles/PMC3743734/

Lee, H., H. Park, E. Ha, YC Hong, M. Ha, H. Park, BN Kim, B. Lee, SJ Lee, KY Lee, JH Kim, KS Jeong, and Y. Kim. "Effect of Breastfeeding Duration on Cognitive Development in Infants: 3-Year Follow-up Study." NCBI. April 2016. Accessed October 01, 2017. https://www.ncbi.nlm.nih.gov/pmc/articles/PMC4810341/.

Lerchbaum, E., and B. Obermayer-Pietsch. "Vitamin D and fertility: a systematic review." NCBI. May 2012. Accessed September 24, 2017. https://www.ncbi.nlm.nih.gov/pubmed/22275473.

Lerchbaum, E., and T. Rabe. "Vitamin D and female fertility." NCBI. June 2014. Accessed September 24, 2017. https://www.ncbi.nlm.nih.gov/pubmed/24717915.

Liu, J., P. Leung, and A. Yang. "Breastfeeding and Active Bonding Protects against Children's Internalizing Behavior Problems." NCBI. January 2014. Accessed October 01, 2017. https://www.ncbi.nlm.nih.gov/pmc/articles/PMC3916850/.

Mahon, P., N. Harvey, S. Crozier, H. Inskip, S. Robinson, N. Arden, R. Swaminatham, C. Cooper, and K. Godfrey. "Low maternal vitamin D status and fetal bone development: cohort study." NCBI. January 2010. Accessed September 11, 2017. https://www.ncbi.nlm.nih.gov/pmc/articles/PMC4768344/.

Malekinejad, Hassan, and Aysa Rezabakhsh. "Hormones in Dairy Foods and Their Impact on Public Health - A Narrative Review Article." NCBI. June 2015. Accessed August 30, 2017. https://www.ncbi.nlm.nih.gov/pmc/articles/PMC4524299/.

Mayurama, K., T. Oshima, and K. Ohyama. "Exposure to exogenous estrogen through intake of commercial milk produced from pregnant cows." NCBI. February 2010. Accessed September 10, 2017. https://www.ncbi.nlm.nih.gov/pubmed/19496976.

Michaëlsson, K., A. Wolk, S. Langenskiöld, S. Basu, E. Warensjö Lemming, H. Melhus, and L. Byberg. "Milk intake and risk of mortality and fractures in women and men: cohort studies." NCBI. October 28, 2014. Accessed September 20, 2017. https://www.ncbi.nlm.nih.gov/pubmed/25352269.

Morse, NL. "Benefits of Docosahexaenoic Acid, Folic Acid, Vitamin D and Iodine on Foetal and Infant Brain Development and Function Following Maternal Supplementation during Pregnancy and Lactation." NCBI. July 2017. Accessed September 29, 2017. https://www.ncbi.nlm.nih.gov/pmc/articles/PMC3407995/.

Morton, S., R. Saraf, D. Bandara, K. Bartholomew, C. Gilchrist, P. Atatoa Carr, L. Baylis, C. Wall, H. Blacklock, M. Tebbutt, and C. Grant. "Maternal and perinatal predictors of newborn iron status." New Zealand Medical Journal. September 12, 2014. Accessed September 13, 2017. https://www.nzma.org.nz/journal/read-the-journal/all-issues/2010-2019/2014/vol-127-no-1402/6293.

Nadjarzadeh, A., R. Dehghani Firouzabadi, N. Vazini, H. Daneshbodi, M. Lotfi, and H. Mozaffari-Khosravi. "The effect of omega-3 supplementation on androgen profile and menstrual status in women with polycystic ovary syndrome: A randomized clinical trial." NCBI. August 2013. Accessed September 19, 2017. https://www.ncbi.nlm.nih.gov/pmc/articles/PMC3941370/.

National Institute of Mental Health, "Postpartum Depression Facts." Accessed September 10, 2017 from https://www.nimh.nih.gov/health/publications/postpartum-depression-facts/index.shtml.

Nazni, P. "Association of western diet & lifestyle with decreased fertility." NCBI. November 2014. Accessed September 11, 2017. https://www.ncbi.nlm.nih.gov/pmc/articles/PMC4345758/.

Nelson, Michael. "Vitamin A, liver consumption, and risk of birth defects." NCBI. November 24, 1990. Accessed October 01, 2017. https://www.ncbi.nlm.nih.gov/pmc/articles/PMC1664333/pdf/bmj00207-0012.pdf.

Obeid, R., W. Holzgreve, and K. Pietrzik. "Is 5-methyltetrahydrofolate an alternative to folic acid for the prevention of neural tube defects?" NCBI. September 01, 2013. Accessed September 11, 2017. https://www.ncbi.nlm.nih.gov/pubmed/23482308.

O'Neil, Adrienne, Catherine Itsiopoulos, Helen Skouteris, Rachelle S. Opie, Skye McPhie, Briony Hill, and Felice N. Jacka. "Preventing mental health problems in offspring by targeting dietary intake of pregnant women." BMC Medicine. November 14, 2014. Accessed September 13, 2017. https://bmcmedicine.biomedcentral.com/articles/10.1186/s12916-014-0208-0.

Pase, CS, K. Roversi, F. Trevisol, FT Kuhn, AJ Schuster, LT Vey, VT Dias, RC Barcelos, J. Piccolo, T. Emanuelli, and ME Burger. "Influence of perinatal trans fat on behavioral responses and brain oxidative status of adolescent rats acutely exposed to stress." NCBI. September 05, 2013. Accessed September 02, 2017. https://www.ncbi.nlm.nih.gov/pubmed/23742847.

Qiu, C., KB Coughlin, IO Frederick, TK Sorensen, and MA Williams. "Dietary fiber intake in early pregnancy and risk of subsequent preeclampsia." NCBI. August 2008. Accessed September 19, 2017. https://www.ncbi.nlm.nih.gov/pubmed/18636070.

Rapley, G., and T. Murkett. *Baby-Led Weaning: The Essential Guide to Introducing Solid Foods*. New York, NY: Workman Publishing, 2010.

Rivellese, AA, DE Natale, and S. Lilli. "Type of dietary fat and insulin resistance." NCBI. June 2002. Accessed September 20, 2017. https://www.ncbi.nlm.nih.gov/pubmed/12079860.

Rombaldi Bernardi, J., R. De Souza Escobar, C. Francisco Ferreira, and P. Pelufo Silveira. "Fetal and Neonatal Levels of Omega-3: Effects on Neurodevelopment, Nutrition, and Growth." NCBI. October 17, 2017. Accessed September 24, 2017. https://www.ncbi.nlm.nih.gov/pmc/articles/PMC3483668/.

Sadeghi, A., S. Shahrokh, and M. Reza Zali. "An unusual cause of constipation in a patient without any underlying disorders." NCBI. February 19, 2015. Accessed September 10, 2017. https://www.ncbi.nlm.nih.gov/pmc/articles/PMC4403030/.

Saldeen, P., and T. Saldeen. "Women and omega-3 Fatty acids." NCBI. October 2004. Accessed September 19, 2017. https://www.ncbi.nlm.nih.gov/pubmed/15385858.

Savage, Jennifer, Jennifer Orlet Fisher, and Leann Birch. "Parental Influence on Eating Behavior." NCBI. March 02, 2007. Accessed September 01, 2017. https://www.ncbi.nlm.nih.gov/pmc/articles/PMC2531152/

Scaglione, F., and G. Panzavolta. "Folate, folic acid and 5-methyltetrahydrofolate are not the same thing." NCBI. May 2014. Accessed September 05, 2017. https://www.ncbi.nlm.nih.gov/pubmed/24494987.

Scholl, TO. "Iron status during pregnancy: setting the stage for mother and infant." NCBI. May 2005. Accessed September 29, 2017. https://www.ncbi.nlm.nih.gov/pubmed/15883455.

Scott, J., C. Binns, K. Graham, and W. Oddy. "Predictors of the early introduction of solid foods in infants: results of a cohort study." NCBI. September 22, 2009. Accessed September 29, 2017. https://www.ncbi.nlm.nih.gov/pmc/articles/PMC2754451/.

Seligman, PA, JH Caskey, JL Frazier, RM Zucker, ER Podell, and RH Allen. "Measurements of iron absorption from prenatal multivitamin—mineral supplements." NCBI. March 1983. Accessed September 05, 2017. https://www.ncbi.nlm.nih.gov/pubmed/6823378.

Sharma, A., S. Amarnath, M. Thulasimani, and S. Ramaswamy. "Artificial sweeteners as a sugar substitute: Are they really safe?" NCBI. May 2016. Accessed September 24, 2017. https://www.ncbi.nlm.nih.gov/pmc/articles/PMC4899993/.

Sharts-Hopko, NC. "Oral intake during labor: a review of the evidence." NCBI. July 2010. Accessed September 29, 2017. https://www.ncbi.nlm.nih.gov/pubmed/20585208.

Singata, M., J. Tranmer, and G. Gyte. "Eating and drinking in labour." NCBI. August 22, 2013. Accessed September 29, 2017. https://www.ncbi.nlm.nih.gov/pubmedhealth/PMH0012411/.

Singh, M. "Essential fatty acids, DHA and human brain." NCBI. March 01, 2005. Accessed September 05, 2017. https://www.ncbi.nlm.nih.gov/pubmed/15812120.

Sonagra, A., S. Biradar, and J. Murthy. "Normal Pregnancy- A State of Insulin Resistance." Normal Pregnancy- A State of Insulin Resistance. November 2014. Accessed September 10, 2017. https://www.ncbi.nlm.nih.gov/pmc/articles/PMC4290225/.

Sperling, JD, JD Dahlke, and BM Sibai. "Restriction of oral intake during labor: whither are we bound?" NCBI. May 2016. Accessed September 29, 2017. https://www.ncbi.nlm.nih.gov/pubmed/26812080.

Stuebe, A. "The Risks of Not Breastfeeding for Mothers and Infants." NCBI. 2009. Accessed October 01, 2017. https://www.ncbi.nlm.nih.gov/pmc/articles/PMC2812877/.

Swithers, S. "Artificial sweeteners produce the counterintuitive effect of inducing metabolic derangements." NCBI. September 2013. Accessed September 24, 2017. https://www.ncbi.nlm.nih.gov/pmc/articles/PMC3772345/.

Tolkien, Z., L. Stecher, and J. Powell. "Ferrous Sulfate Supplementation Causes Significant Gastrointestinal Side-Effects in Adults: A Systematic Review and Meta-Analysis." NCBI. February 20, 2015. Accessed September 06, 2017. https://www.ncbi.nlm.nih.gov/pmc/articles/PMC4336293/pdf/pone.0117383.pdf.

Tripkovic, L., H. Lambert, K. Hart, C. Smith, G. Bucca, S. Penson, G. Chope, and E. Hypponen. "Comparison of vitamin D2 and vitamin D3 supplementation in raising serum 25-hydroxyvitamin D status: a systematic review and meta-analysis1,2,3." NCBI. May 02, 2012. Accessed September 05, 2017. https://www.ncbi.nlm.nih.gov/pmc/articles/PMC3349454/#!po=78.1250

Urrutia, R., and J. Thorp. "Vitamin D in Pregnancy: Current Concepts." NCBI. March 2012. Accessed September 11, 2017. https://www.ncbi.nlm.nih.gov/pmc/articles/PMC3709246/.

Vennemann, MM, T. Bajanowski, B. Brinkmann, G. Jorch, K. Yücesan, C. Sauerland, and EA Mitchell. "Does breastfeeding reduce the risk of sudden infant death syndrome?" NCBI. March 2009. Accessed October 01, 2017. https://www.ncbi.nlm.nih.gov/pubmed/19254976.

Von Ehrenstein, OS, H. Aralis, ME Flores, and B. Ritz. "Fast food consumption in pregnancy and subsequent asthma symptoms in young children." NCBI. September 26, 2015. Accessed September 01, 2017. https://www.ncbi.nlm.nih.gov/pubmed/26109272.

Wei, SQ. "Vitamin D and pregnancy outcomes." NCBI. December 2014. Accessed September 27, 2017. https://www.ncbi.nlm.nih.gov/pubmed/25310531.

"Why can't we give water to a breastfeeding baby before the 6 months, even when it is hot?" World Health Organization. July 2014. Accessed September 29, 2017. http://www.who.int/features/qa/breastfeeding/en/.

Winchester, Paul, Cathy Proctor, and Jun Ying. "County-level pesticide use and risk of shortened gestation and preterm birth." NCBI. November 23, 2015. Accessed September 01, 2017. https://www.ncbi.nlm.nih.gov/pmc/articles/PMC5067698/pdf/APA-105-e107.pdf.

Wojcicki, J., and MB Heyman. "Maternal omega-3 fatty acid supplementation and risk for perinatal maternal depression." NCBI. May 2011. Accessed September 29, 2017. https://www.ncbi.nlm.nih.gov/pmc/articles/PMC3119925/.

Zeisel, SH. "Nutritional importance of choline for brain development." NCBI. December 2004. Accessed September 29, 2017. https://www.ncbi.nlm.nih.gov/pubmed/15640516.

Zhao, Xin , Rui Fang, Renqiang Yu, Daozhen Chen, Jun Zhao, and Jianping Xiao. "Maternal Vitamin D Status in the Late Second Trimester and the Risk of Severe Preeclampsia in Southeastern China." NCBI. February 14, 2017. Accessed August 30, 2017. https://www.ncbi.nlm.nih.gov/pmc/articles/PMC5331569/.

Ziegler, EE. "Adverse effects of cow's milk in infants." NCBI. 2007. Accessed September 30, 2017. https://www.ncbi.nlm.nih.gov/pubmed/17664905.

Ziegler, EE. "Consumption of cow's milk as a cause of iron deficiency in infants and toddlers." NCBI. November 2011. Accessed September 10, 2017. https://www.ncbi.nlm.nih.gov/pubmed/22043881.

Acknowledgments

There are so many people who made *The Whole Food Pregnancy Plan* possible, but it would have never come to life if it were not for my husband, Richard, and my son, Alex. Without my husband, I would have never become so passionate about nutrition, and of course, I am a mother because of him. Thank you, Richard, for teaching me so much and for being an undying source of support, not only for this book but also in raising our beautiful boy.

To my parents, Steve and Norma—thank you for always backing me in everything I do.

My brother, Steven, and his fiancé, Jennifer—thank you for the encouragement and for the opportunity to work with Modesto Junior College and the women's soccer team.

To my father- and mother-in-law, Rich and Dorothy Oliva and the rest of the Oliva family in Ohio, Texas, and Florida, for always rooting me on.

My agent, Pamela Harty, I cannot thank you enough for believing in this project from day one.

To Leah Zarra and Skyhorse, I truly appreciate all of your help and this opportunity.

To Dr. Kenneth Akey, your support with this project and the care you have provided our son means the world to us.

To Katie Williams, Kara Cruz, and Nadine Grzeskowiak, thank you for contributing your expertise to this project—it has been a pleasure working with you all.

My wonderful friends, Maxine Goynes, Lara Drew-Aktary, Alicia Pasquini, Andrea Cardoza, Madeline Hill, Deanna Molina, Sabrina Parenti, Stephanie Johnston, and Bridget Pizzo, for offering unlimited advice, support, and reassurance through this journey.

Priscila Sobrero, Dawn Costello, and Sabryna Costello, Alex's adored babysitters, thank you all for taking excellent care of our boy during days/evenings when I was writing.

To my doula, Lauren Jacobs of Doulas of Orange County, your knowledge and assistance has been invaluable.

And to my incredible food photography team, Alan De Herrera, Chef Elizabeth Whitt, and food stylist, Judean Sakimoto—I had a blast with you all.

About the Author

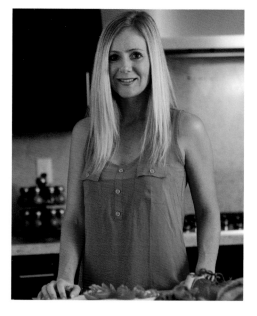

Aimee Aristotelous, co-author of *The Eat to Keep Fit Diet*, is a certified nutritionist, specializing in prenatal dietetics. Aristotelous provides weekly fitness and nutrition tips to her 22,000 Facebook followers and has been the exclusive nutritionist for NBC affiliate KSEE 24 News in Fresno, California, appearing in more than fifty nutrition and cooking segments. She has six years of nutrition consulting experience and has helped more than 2,000 people lose weight and get healthy! Aimee's interest in nutrition began as she struggled with her own weight gain after taking a sedentary office job in her twenties once her athletic career came to an end. She furthered her nutrition education in prenatal dietetics after learning she was pregnant, as she witnessed the prevalence of diet-related pregnancy ailments amongst her peers. A California native, Aimee currently resides in Fort Lauderdale, Florida, with her husband and son, and enjoys the beach, cooking, and traveling.

Aimee used her own gluten-free pregnancy as a platform to apply her educational background and research, which resulted in an optimally healthy, active, and ideal pregnancy. With a twenty-five-pound total weight gain, and a 9 pound, 12 ounce baby boy, she recovered to her pre-pregnancy weight of 125 pounds before her six-week doctor's clearance to return to exercise. During her ninth month of pregnancy, she was hired by the company "Belly Bandit" to model a line of their pregnancy lingerie. In addition to her Nutrition and Wellness certification through American Fitness Professionals and Associates, Aimee has a bachelor's degree in business/marketing from California State University, Long Beach. She has ten years of professional marketing experience for a large, private California-based company.

Contributing Writers

Dr. Kenneth Akey, MD

Dr. Kenneth Akey, MD, FAAP, is a board certified pediatric doctor who serves Georgia's Newnan and Coweta Counties. During more than twenty-five years of private practice (many of which were based in Orange County, California), he has cultivated many strong relationships with his patients and their families. Dr. Akey's passions include developmental pediatrics and nutrition. He stresses the importance of a healthy diet to all of his patients and their parents, as they are often the ones with ultimate control over what their child eats. When Dr. Akey isn't

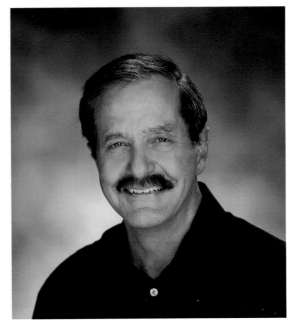

providing warm, knowledgeable care for children, he enjoys working out, being involved at his church, and spending time with his wife, children, and grandchildren.

Nadine Grzeskowiak RN, BSN, CEN

Nadine Grzeskowiak, RN, BSN, CEN began her nursing career in 1992 in emergency, trauma, and critical care at hospitals throughout Oregon. In 2006, she was diagnosed with celiac disease—at the time of diagnosis, she expected to be dead in six months or less. Within two weeks of beginning a gluten-free diet, her health began to improve remarkably which led to a life and career-changing shift. Nadine founded three nursing businesses shortly thereafter: RN on Call, Inc. in February 2007, Gluten Free RN in March 2007, followed by Celiac Nurse Consulting. Presently Nadine is an expert consultant, author, and professional speaker on all aspects of gluten intolerance and celiac disease, having presented over 1,800 lectures to various audiences. Nadine's first book, *DOUGH NATION: A Nurse's Memoir of Celiac Disease from Missed Diagnosis to Food and Health Activism* was officially released September 2015. In her spare time Nadine can be found climbing mountains, hiking, reading, knitting, and eating excellent meals with family and friends.

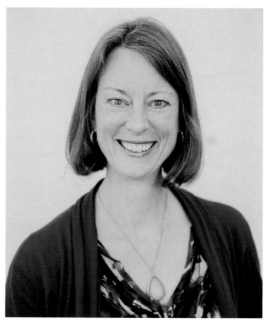

Amanda Long/Amanda Photographic

Katie Munday Williams, RN, BSN, PHN

Katie Munday Williams graduated from the Johns Hopkins School of Nursing in 2004 and has thirteen years of experience in pediatrics and perinatal nursing Her passion is educating parents and families on ways to get the most out of their parenting relationship. She is currently working in public health and plans to finish her lactation consultant certification in 2018. Katie owns BabyMuse Sleep Consulting, which helps parents establish healthy sleep habits for their children using gentle, evidence-based methods. She is also the Co-coordinator for the Nursing Mothers Counsel (Santa Cruz County), offering free breastfeeding peer support to moms and their babies. Katie lives in Santa Cruz,

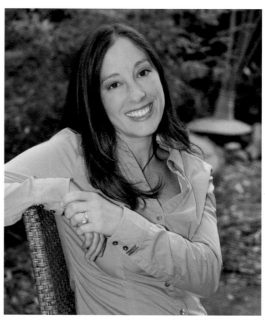

Photo credit: Candy Cooper/Candy Coated Photography

California, with her husband Aaron, daughter Rose, and son James, where they enjoy gawking at whales and building sand castles.

Kara Danielle Cruz, MA, Registered Associate Marriage and Family Therapist

Kara is registered in California as an Associate Marriage and Family Therapist and is employed by a nonprofit organization as a Behavioral Health Clinician, providing individual and family therapy to children and adolescents. Kara works primarily with youth who are experiencing behavioral health diagnoses including neurodevelopmental disorders, anxiety, depression, trauma, and disruptive, impulse control, and conduct disorders. Kara has more than sixteen years' experience working within the educational and human service fields, and is a professional member of the California Association of Marriage and Family Therapists. She received a Bachelor of Arts Degree in Psychology from Chapman

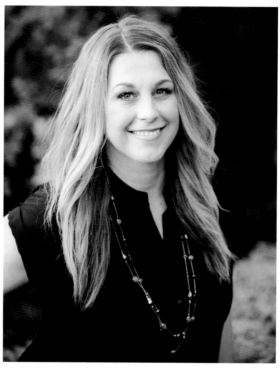

Photo credit: Sara Malough/Plain Jane Photography

University and a Master of Arts Degree in Psychology with an emphasis in Marriage and Family Therapy from Brandman University. In addition to her work with youth and families, Kara has the desire to learn about the connection of physical health and wellness to behavioral health. Kara spends her time away from work with her husband, Alex, and son, Clark, in Central Valley, California.

Conversion Charts

Metric and Imperial Conversions

(These conversions are rounded for convenience)

Ingredient	Cups/Tablespoons/Teaspoons	Ounces	Grams/Milliliters
Butter	1 cup/16 tablespoons/2 sticks	8 ounces	230 grams
Cheese, shredded	1 cup	4 ounces	110 grams
Cream cheese	1 tablespoon	0.5 ounce	14.5 grams
Cornstarch	1 tablespoon	0.3 ounce	8 grams
Flour, all-purpose	1 cup/1 tablespoon	4.5 ounces/0.3 ounce	125 grams/8 grams
Flour, whole wheat	1 cup	4 ounces	120 grams
Fruit, dried	1 cup	4 ounces	120 grams
Fruits or veggies, chopped	1 cup	5 to 7 ounces	145 to 200 grams
Fruits or veggies, puréed	1 cup	8.5 ounces	245 grams
Honey, maple syrup, or corn syrup	1 tablespoon	0.75 ounce	20 grams
Liquids: cream, milk, water, or juice	1 cup	8 fluid ounces	240 milliliters
Oats	1 cup	5.5 ounces	150 grams
Salt	1 teaspoon	0.2 ounce	6 grams
Spices: cinnamon, cloves, ginger, or nutmeg (ground)	1 teaspoon	0.2 ounce	5 milliliters
Sugar, brown, firmly packed	1 cup	7 ounces	200 grams
Sugar, white	1 cup/1 tablespoon	7 ounces/0.5 ounce	200 grams/12.5 grams
Vanilla extract	1 teaspoon	0.2 ounce	4 grams

Oven Temperatures

Fahrenheit	Celsius	Gas Mark
225°	110°	1/4
250°	120°	1/2
275°	140°	1
300°	150°	2
325°	160°	3
350°	180°	4
375°	190°	5
400°	200°	6
425°	220°	7
450°	230°	8

Index